COLD and FLU

HOW to PREVENT it or GET RID of it FAST!

*Use nature's pharmacy to boost your immune system
and stay well all year round.*

By Carol Perkins, N.D., Health Coach

www.natural-choices.info

This book is available in print and ebook at most online retailers.

Disclaimer:

This book contains educational advice and information relating to health care. The Food & Drug Administration has not evaluated these statements. It is not intended to replace medical advice and should be used to supplement rather than replace regular care by your health care practitioner, especially if you are pregnant, nursing, diabetic, or taking medications that could have potential drug interactions.

All efforts have been made to ensure the accuracy of the information contained in this book as of the date of publication. Carol Perkins, N.D. disclaims all liability for any medical outcome that may occur as a result of applying the methods suggested in this book.

Table of Contents

Introduction

As a naturopathic doctor for the past 15 years, one of my greatest passions is to help people reach their highest life potential.

My family has been my greatest motivator to seek solutions to various health concerns from viral infections to cancer. My husband Chris, children Sherry, Deidra and Chris, grandchildren Amanda, Joshua, Alyssa, Julia, Ryan, Adam and Logan have inspired me to educate others to aspire to optimal health and wellness.

Before becoming a naturopathic doctor, I spent nearly 20 years in the computer science field designing and implementing robotics in various parts of the world. Success in this field depends on one's ability to develop methods of *critical thinking*.

This critical thinking has influenced my approach to a patient's health concerns.

I can use logic and reasoning to identify the *root cause* of their illness and then design the best protocol for them to attain optimal health.

Ignore your health and it will go away.
Prevention and optimum health requires a good
"Health Coach".

Flu is one of the most notorious diseases mankind has had to face. We can expect it to come every year giving a quick, mild course or be a real threat. It is not the disease itself, but the possible complications such as pneumonia that make it dangerous. Flu and colds can be mild or truly debilitating, taking its toll for days or even weeks, especially when it is out of control. Since flu and colds are expected, you can prepare yourself and your family for it throughout the year - *if* you have adequate information and tools.

To be ready for this year's flu and cold attacks, it is absolutely critical that you maintain a healthy diet, get a moderate amount of exercise and support your immune system.

If the prevention plan fails and you do not escape symptoms of flu and cold, then options exist to shorten its course and prevent further complications. But first, you must be able to distinguish whether your symptoms are from the flu or cold. They share some similar symptoms but the course of disease is vastly different. A cold rarely leaves you bedridden, while the flu can easily do that – sometimes for a long time. This is especially important in the case of children whose immune systems may not be well developed enough to resist disease.

The universal fact is that nature is your best pharmacy.

This includes nutritious foods, herbal remedies, homeopathy, and just good common sense. In this book, you will find concise, yet clear and useful advice on how to stop flu and cold from ruining your precious time.

The book is divided into 4 main parts:
1. Why do we get sick?
2. Disease PREVENTION strategies.
3. Acute infection plan.
4. Chronic infections and "cytokine storm" recommendations.

Chapter 1: Why do we get sick?

Despite modern medical care in the United States, disease rates are increasing. Obesity, diabetes, autoimmune diseases and cancer are on the rise.

So what is the problem?

I believe that doctors do not focus on the *"root" causes* of why people are getting sick. Our health care model needs to be *patient-oriented rather than disease-oriented*.

According to 2014 statistics reported by the Center for Disease Control (CDC):

- 9.3% of the U.S. population is diabetic – an increase from 6 million to 16 million in the last 15 years. Another 21 million have "impaired glucose tolerance".

- 35.7% of adults and 17% of children and adolescents are obese. On average, obese people have medical costs that are $1429 more than medical costs of normal weight people per year. In fact, the U.S. has the highest obesity rate in the world.

- Some form of depression, anxiety, or fatigue affects over 50% of the U.S. population.

Robyn O'Brien, the author of *AllergyKids*, states the following statistics:

- 400% increase in foods allergies
- 300% increase in asthma
- 1,000 – 6,000% increase in autism
- 400% increase in ADHD
- 400% increase in Celiac disease
- 45% of children will be insulin dependent in 10 years

Pretty Scary!

There is a lot of human misery reflected in these frightening statistics, plus billions of dollars involved in the health care needs these people require. Many decision makers in America continue to claim that the United States has the greatest health care system in the world.

But the fact is that America spends over 16% of its gross domestic product (GDP) on health care. Compare this with similar nations like Japan, Australia, Canada, and rich European nations who spend between 8 to 11% of their GDP on health care.

Would you be surprised if I told you that Americans, the citizens of the wealthiest country in the world, have a lower life expectancy rate, higher rate of heart disease and cancer, and an infant mortality rate that is twice as high as many other rich industrialized nations?

Do you think improving public health policies is the answer?

The more realistic answer, in my opinion, is proper nutrition, exercise and taking control of toxins in our environment, for a start. Even the National Institute of Health agrees when it states that four of the six leading causes of death in the U. S. are linked to unhealthy diets.

Health care spending is expected to reach nearly 20% of America's GDP within the next 10 years, which is unsustainable.

The cost of prescription drugs is rising even faster than the general rise in health care costs. In fact, drug companies currently have a reputation of being "Pill Pushers" – creating a demand for pills where there is not even a disease.

The fear of being sued leads doctors to practice "defensive medicine," i.e., ordering excessive tests, avoiding risky procedures and referring patients to see other expert doctors. This kind of "defensive medicine" is becoming routine, leading to higher costs in health care and a waste of the American health care system's resources.

So why are Americans so sick?

There are many reasons for this. Let's start with food allergies/intolerances: Why are so many children being diagnosed with food allergies/intolerances?

Consider the following facts about food allergies/intolerances:

- Food allergies/intolerances result in an elevated *CORTISOL* (a stress hormone) as the immune system reacts to allergens released from the gut into the blood where it should not be. This is a *constant low level of stress*.
- Elevated cortisol results in elevated *INSULIN*. Cortisol and Insulin work together - insulin is the buffer for cortisol.

- Constant elevated insulin leads to *INSULIN RESISTANCE* and *STORAGE OF FAT*, which eventually leads to diabetes, obesity and other degenerative diseases, if it is not reversed.

Dr. Mark Hyman claims that our modern wheat may be driving people to obesity, diabetes, heart disease, cancer, etc.

Dr. Hyman's research shows that new, modern wheat *looks* like wheat but contains super-starch called amylopectin A that is **super-fattening**. But it makes fluffy products!

Modern wheat also contains super-gluten that is **super-inflammatory**.

Another surprising thing - modern wheat contains forms of **super-drugs** that are **super-addictive** and makes you crave it and eat more. How is this possible? Exorphins created from polypeptides in wheat bind to opioid receptors in the brain.

Possible symptoms of wheat sensitivity and/or allergy include bloating, gas, diarrhea, nausea, indigestion, abdominal pain, constipation, low appetite, vomiting, etc.

Due to malabsorption of nutrients, over time other symptoms may occur such as depression, fatigue, delayed growth in children, hair loss, itchy skin, mouth ulcers, joint pain, seizures, tingling/numbness in extremities, irritable/fussy behavior, headaches, migraines, compromised immune system and much more.

Environmental Toxins

In our industrialized environment, we are constantly exposed to xenoestrogens - chemicals that provoke or mimic estrogen in the body. Examples of common xenoestrogens include phthalates, pesticides and Bisphenol A (BPA).

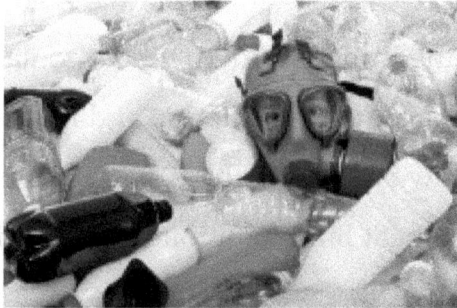

Phthalates are found in plastics and cosmetics. Pesticides are often used on fruits and vegetables. Furthermore, the use of hand sanitizers and creams were found to increase absorption of BPA into the system.

**Unfortunately, xenoestrogens are everywhere
in our modern world.**

These xenoestrogens mimic estrogen and disrupt normal functions in the body leading to damage of the reproductive system and other organs and can even promote cancer. Simply put, xenoestrogens contribute to "estrogen dominance."
In men, this can lead to feminizing qualities, reduce sperm count and increase cancer risk. In women, it can induce early puberty and menstrual abnormalities, and also increase cancer risk.

Children are very vulnerable since xenoestrogens can be passed from the mother to the fetus; or these substances can be transferred to babies when they come in contact with adults wearing cosmetics that contain xenoestrogens.

Lack of adequate sleep can affect the immune system.

Stress is a big factor.

Chronic stress has reached epidemic proportions in Western culture. In response to stress, the hormone *cortisol* is released into the system causing suppression of body functions such as digestion and immune activity.

Excess sugar intake can reduce the ability of white blood cells of the immune system to kill invaders.

Even worse, the immune-suppressing effect of sugar starts immediately after ingestion. For example, a can of soda contains about nine teaspoons of sugar. This can suppress the immune system by 30% for three hours. So cutting out excess sugar is a very important step to support immunity.

Excessive alcohol can put the immune system at risk.

Alcoholic beverages deprive the body of protective nutrients, suppresses the availability of white blood cells to multiply, and inhibits the action of natural killer cells.

Processed foods, artificial flavors, colors, dyes and sweeteners can decrease immunity and increase susceptibility to illness.

About 40 years ago, food processing manufacturers discovered that a food's shelf life could be extended by destroying its enzymes. The problem with this is that enzymes in foods also help digest the food. Thus, when you eat processed food, it is partially digested. This partially digested food enters the bloodstream where the immune system perceives it as the enemy and then attacks it (food allergy).

So why are people getting sicker?

We spend more money on health care than ever before. We take more drugs than ever before, yet we are sicker than ever before in history. Over the years, the pharmaceutical industry has come up with different theories about why people get sick.

Bacteria?
Viruses?
Genetics?

First, it was *bacteria* and germs. The super wonder drug of the day was antibiotics, touted to eliminate disease forever and cure all illness and disease. That theory has proved to be wrong. Stronger and stronger antibiotics have been developed. Yet people continue to get sicker and sicker.

The next theory was that *viruses* were the cause of all illness and disease. It is a fact that antibiotics have no effect on viruses even though doctors prescribe them for practically everything. Our government estimates that half of the 100 million antibiotic prescriptions written each year are totally unnecessary.

The current theory of the day is that all sickness, disease, and illness is caused by *genetic defects*. Of course, the only answer to this is more drugs. We hear it every day:

"You're overweight because you have a genetic defect, and a drug is being worked on that can solve that genetic defect to make you thin."

"Diabetes is nothing more than genetics, so we'll work on a drug that will correct that genetic disposition and solve the problem."

Think about this: Would a particular drug be needed if a cure was found for a certain disease? How would that affect the profits made by the drug companies?

In a medical emergency, drugs and surgery can save your life. But the *"root cause"* of symptoms are rarely addressed.

What about all the drugs that were "proven" safe and effective by the FDA and years later "proven" to be dangerous and taken off the market.

And now, drugs are being advertised on the TV, radio, newspapers, magazines, etc. - all in an attempt to evoke certain emotions in you so you feel that you need that drug. What baffles me is why someone would actually take a drug after hearing all the side effects from it. But these drug advertisements are amazingly effective.

Another interesting fact is this: the FDA has set as law that no natural remedy can be claimed to prevent or treat a disease (only a drug can be used to claim this). Why? Part of the reason is that there is insufficient research on natural remedies but another reason could be that natural remedies cannot be patented so there is no substantial monetary gain.

<u>**So why do you get sick?**</u>
Is it Bacteria?
Viruses?
Genetics?

Well, let's think about it.
You don't catch cancer. Your body develops cancer.
You don't catch diabetes. Your body develops it.
You don't catch obesity. Your body becomes obese.
You don't catch acid reflux. It's developed.

These are conditions that are developed in the body. You don't catch them.

The majority of illness is, in fact, <u>self-inflicted</u>.

The question remains - Why do we get sick? There are 3 reasons:

Toxic load.

Biochemical individuality – each of us is unique.

Health care is disease-focused rather than patient-focused.

Let's start with a story about the first reason - *toxic load*.

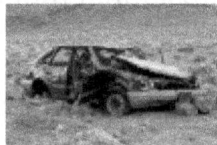

As a man drove through the mountains one day, he stopped now and then to load rocks into the trunk of his car. With each new rock, his car got slower and slower and sagged lower and lower until all of a sudden - BAMMM!!!--his suspension gave way. The gas tank slammed to the ground, sparks flew, and gasoline ignited. By this time, there was nothing left of the man's car but twisted metal and smoking ashes.

Many people are like that man's car. They go through life accumulating various kinds of "rocks" (or toxic stressors), knowingly or not, that place a growing burden on the body's ability to function normally.

In other words, anything that taxes the normal functioning of your body and pushes you away from optimal health can be referred to as a toxin.

Along the road of life the total load of toxic stressors can become too much. Physical breakdown occurs. A major health crisis sets in - cancer and other degenerative conditions like heart attack, stroke, diabetes, Alzheimer's, multiple sclerosis, chronic fatigue syndrome, arthritis, allergies, and many, many other such crisis's.

The body's various systems become compromised because there are too many "rocks" in the trunk. You may be able to handle *some* of the toxic stressors, but as they pile up, eventually your body can't keep pulling the load.

The picture below illustrates the process of going down the stairs from optimal health to declining health. At the top half of the stairs are signs of health. At the bottom half of the stairs are signs of disease.

But, also notice that the reverse is possible – climbing the stairs from declining health back to optimal health.

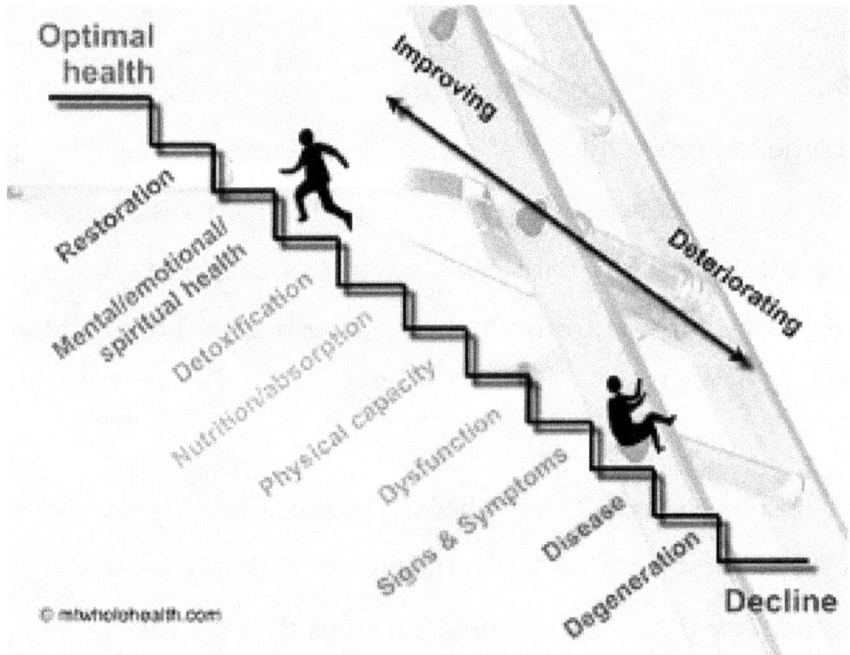

Optimal health

Improving

Deteriorating

Restoration

Mental/emotional/ spiritual health

Detoxification

Nutrition/absorption

Physical capacity

Dysfunction

Signs & Symptoms

Disease

Degeneration

Decline

© mtwholehealth.com

The 8 Laws of Health

To correct the "root cause" of disease, one must first find the area(s) of imbalance and dysfunction in the body, typically from one or more of the following 8 Laws of Health:

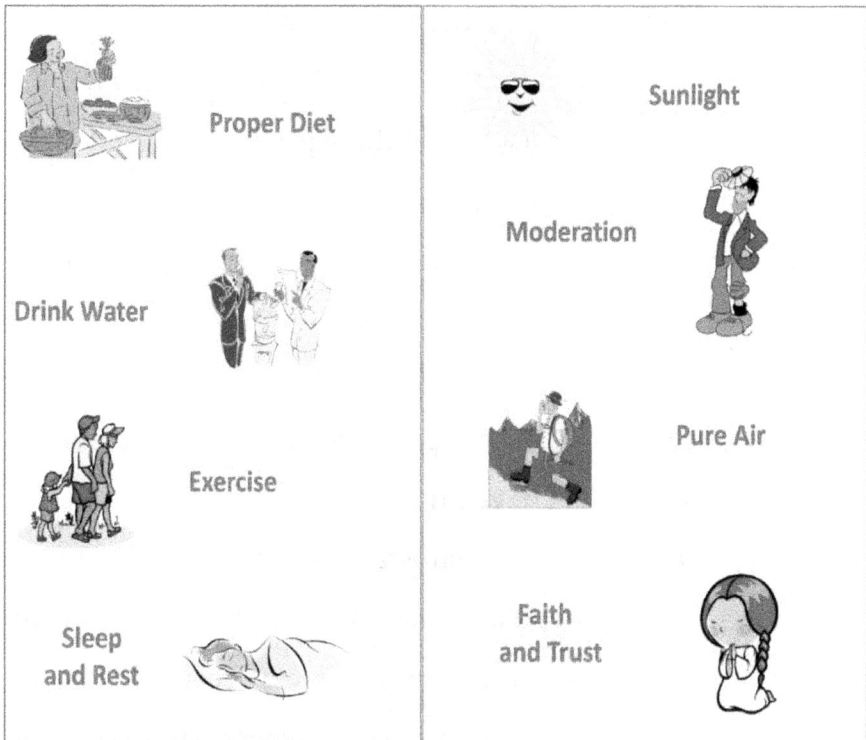

Proper Diet

Drink Water

Exercise

Sleep and Rest

Sunlight

Moderation

Pure Air

Faith and Trust

This is what I tell my patients:

Unless you have a diet and lifestyle that supports health,
then all the medications, supplements, and exercise
in the world will not provide what you need
for optimal health in a simple way.

There are no shortcuts to optimal health. You must start with diet and lifestyle. The challenge of eating well is to choose *real* food and ignore the new products introduced each year.

When discussing diet with patients, I sometimes ask them, "What did your grandparents eat on a day-to-day basis?" The responses vary depending on the age of the patient. If they can remember their grandparents' diet before the 1950's, generally it was simple - a whole food blend of meat-potato-vegetables.

"Food scientists" get us to buy products through our taste buds. After all, humans have an inborn preference for sweetness, salt and fat. Thus, substances can be added to products to "addict" unsuspecting consumers so they will buy more and more of these unnatural products. Eventually, many consumers will use food as a form of self-medication to temporarily boost their energy and mood.

The truth is, most American consumers are so addicted to sugar that they will deny their addictions in the same way that a crack or heroin addict might.

For example, if they don't have the sugar fix found in coffee, cereal, donuts, soda, candy, desert, and hidden in processed foods, they can suffer serious withdrawal symptoms and go crazy with moodiness and irritability. They may even become sweaty and light-headed.

I came across this CounterThink cartoon recently:

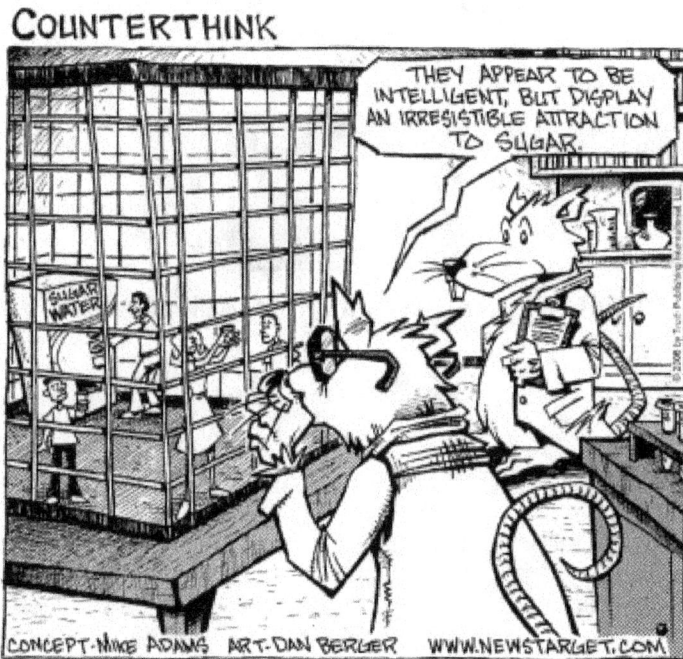

Can you guess what an outside observer would think about our modern addiction to sugar? Yes, they would think humans are strange animals to be so controlled by a crystalline white substance.

Chapter 2: Is disease a friend or an enemy?

DISEASE is the effort of nature to sweep out the dirt brought into the body by our ignorance of the 8 Laws of Health shown previously. A cold virus is a good example of nature trying to sweep the dirt out of the body: The white, yellow or green snot that comes out of the nose and lungs is the dirt or toxins that have piled up in your body.

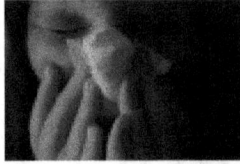

Cold symptoms are an effort to clean house.

You don't *catch* a cold from the air or from someone else. It's because your body is clogged up with sugar, processed foods, excess stress, staying up too late at night, etc.

What can you do to help your body "clean house"? As I stated previously, the first step is to correct the "root cause" by finding the area(s) of imbalance and dysfunction in the body:

Proper Diet

Adequate, clean water

Exercise

Sunlight

Pure air

Sleep and rest

Everything in moderation

Spiritual health

I'm sure you are anxious to get started on this very important topic. But first, I would like to address the questions many people are asking:

> **"With all the information we are bombarded with, who can we believe? Who can we trust?**
>
> **How do I know they are not just trying to sell me something?**
>
> **How are Naturopathic doctors like myself different in their approach to health?**

I intend to answer all three of these questions in the next chapter.

Chapter 3: How are Naturopathic doctors different in their approach to health?

The answer is simple - Naturopathic doctors such as myself, implement the *patient-oriented* rather than the *disease-oriented* health care model. This is an important concept to understand because it goes a long way in finding the "root cause" of disease.

The focus and motivation of Naturopathic doctors is to help patients achieve optimal health and wellness so they no longer need to depend on prescription medications or supplements unless absolutely necessary.

The disease-oriented approach to health care focuses almost entirely on the management of *symptoms* of disease rather than *curing* disease. Of course, treating symptoms can be important – especially when symptoms are a result of acute and/or life-threatening malfunctions. In fact, America probably has the best knowledge and technology for acute care in the world.

A great analogy of the disease-oriented approach to health care is the example that Michael E. Rothman, M.D. gives in his book *Edibolic Stress*. He calls it '**The Car Doctor – Idle Worship**'. Although this example is a bit far-fetched, it will help illustrate how backward it is to treat your symptoms instead of the "root cause."

Imagine you are driving your car, and the car begins to stall every time you slow down and idle. So you bring the vehicle to a mechanic, and instead of doing a diagnostic evaluation, he listens to your car's symptoms and quickly declares, "I believe your car is suffering from **slow idle syndrome**. I can provide a remedy for that." His remedy for slow idle syndrome is to increase the idle speed of your engine and sends you on your way. So now when you are sitting at a red light, the car no longer stalls. However, because the idle speed has been increased, you find that you must constantly hit the brakes to keep the car from going too fast.

You bring the car back to the same mechanic and explain the new problem, to which he states, "It now appears that your car is exhibiting signs of **hypobrakia**. I can alleviate that symptom as well."

He then proceeds to partially apply your parking brake and tells you to drive around with your brakes on. Now your car doesn't stall when you go too slowly and no longer speeds along when you idle, but new difficulties have arisen. You notice that the gas mileage is down, the car is starting to overheat, and the acceleration is poor. Again, you bring your car to the mechanic. This time he states that your poor gas mileage and your poor acceleration are happening because **"your car is getting old."** He recommends temporarily installing a cooling system to lower the engine temperature – while you look for a new car.

You decide to get a second opinion and take your car to another mechanic. He opens up the hood and does a thorough logical analysis of all the systems and components of your vehicle. He discovers that your idle speed is set too high, your parking brake is stuck in the on position, and your car's spark plugs are extremely worn down. In fact, they are so worn that they were the reason your car started stalling initially. He changes the spark plugs, resets the idle speed, releases your parking brake, and now your car works as good as new.

Treating complex medical problems is much more difficult than fixing a malfunctioning car, but the principles are the same. Unfortunately, many people have their systems further disturbed and imbalanced by well-meaning doctors who are focused on treating their symptoms.

Let's take high blood pressure for an example. The most common treatment is a drug that frequently leads to new disturbances to your body and thus new symptoms. Keep in mind that all drugs have side effects because they are toxic to the body. The most common drug that is recommended for high blood pressure is a beta blocker. What does a beta blocker do? It blocks the excitatory hormones (adrenaline and noradrenaline) on the beta-adrenergic receptors to slow your heart down.

So essentially, beta blockers interfere with your "fight or flight" stress response – they slow down the idle speed of your heart. The result can be that the heart can slow down too much and/or the blood pressure can get too low. The person may experience fatigue, fluid buildup, dizziness, foggy thinking, low blood sugar and many more side-effects.
Did the beta blocker fix the original problem? Probably not. But it did lower the blood pressure!

Did it make the patient feel better or reduce the risk for a heart attack or stroke? Probably not. The fact is that beta blockers are known to significantly increase the risk of developing diabetes, weight gain and high triglycerides. These in turn, increase your risk for heart disease!

If your doctor is taking you down this road, it may be time to look for a different health care approach, especially if you have a chronic health concern. Finding the "root cause" and correcting it, is the natural path to optimal health.

How is a *patient-focused* approach different?

A patient-focused approach is based on scientific evidence plus **common sense**. Optimal health depends on a healthy diet, physical activity, lifestyle choices and how well we cope with stress. It's also important to identify and remove barriers to health by creating a healing internal and external environment. A patient-focused approach understands that everyone has a unique mental, physical, emotional, genetic and spiritual makeup. Thus, individualized strategies must be developed for each patient.

Chapter 4: Ways to protect your family

With the kids in school, adults heading indoors as the temperatures cool and the dreaded flu season upon us, thoughts quickly turn to immunity – how to maintain it, boost it and keep it working optimally. But even a typically strong immune system can wither in the face of various infections, especially viral infections. The questions I am asked the most on this subject are the following:

How can I prevent an infection?
If an infection hits, how can I lessen the intensity and severity?
Do I need to get the flu vaccine? Is it safe?
Is the Ebola virus something I should worry about
or is it just media hype?

Keep in mind the following facts: an estimated 80% of flu-like illness reported during the "flu season" is <u>not</u> caused by influenza and most people who are hospitalized or die because of flu complications have pre-existing health conditions or are children with immature immune systems who are unable to mount a strong defense.

The health of your immune system is
the most important aspect of protecting yourself.

To prevent disease, you will need to expand your knowledge of nutrition, lifestyle and natural medicine. Modern medicine's solution to disease is drugs and vaccines. They do not discuss alternative solutions that have been used for generations to prevent disease and save lives.

Natural immune-boosting therapies exist to help protect you from ANY virus.

What about the flu vaccine?

From my observation over the years, those who have gotten flu shots experience colds and flu as much as people who don't get the shot. Moreover, the research I've read clearly indicates that flu shot effectiveness is a pretty dubious proposition, no matter what your doctor says.

Currently, the Ebola virus is in the news and many people are concerned that it will come to America. The only solution offered by our government is the hope for a vaccine.

But the fact is, vaccines MUST be based on the viral code that is circulating in the wild in order to be effective. For example, to make a flu vaccine, the viruses that are circulating in the wild must be used in a weakened state. The problem is that it takes many months to make a vaccine. So the current flu shot that people are getting just protects them from the previous year's virus strain since the virus continually mutates (changes) from year to year.

During the 2012-13 flu season, the CDC gauged the flu vaccine's effectiveness at 56% across all age groups – slightly better odds than tossing a coin!

Another concern is the preservatives and heavy metals added to the flu vaccine that can cause problems in some people. It makes more sense to keep your immune system healthy so it can build its own antibodies naturally. Personally, I am exposed to many sick people but rarely get the flu; and I have never had the flu vaccine. If I get symptoms, I simply boost my immune system and breeze through it.

A healthy immune system will build antibodies naturally!

Is it the flu or is it a cold?

According to the Mayo Clinic, influenza is a viral infection that attacks your respiratory system – nose, throat and lungs. Initially, one may experience cold-like symptoms like runny nose, sneezing and sore throat.

Colds develop slowly, but influenza comes on suddenly. Colds are a nuisance but you feel much worse with flu.

<u>**Common signs and symptoms of flu include:**</u>
- Fever over 100 degrees F (38 degrees C)
- Aching muscles, especially in your back, arms and legs
- Chills and sweats
- Headache
- Dry cough
- Fatigue and weakness
- Nasal congestion

According to the CDC, a number of reports of severe respiratory illness have been reported among young and middle-aged adults, many of whom are infected with influenza A pdm09 (pH1N1) virus.

There have been multiple pH1N1-associated hospitalizations, including many requiring intensive care admission and some fatalities. Flu activity is likely to continue for some time, particularly in parts of the country that are showing recent increases in activity.

The pH1N1 virus that emerged in 2009 caused more illness in children and young adults compared to older adults, although severe illness was seen in all age groups. pH1N1 has been the predominant circulating virus so far.

We can learn from the1918 Spanish flu pandemic.
The most devastating outbreak of disease in history was the 1918 Flu Pandemic, a H1N1 type virus. It spread to nearly every part of the world. In contrast to most influenza outbreaks which affect the elderly, children and immune-compromised persons, most of its victims were healthy, young adults.

By the time the killer virus died out a year later, an estimated 50-100 million people had died world-wide. An estimated 500 million people, one third of the world's population, had become infected.

Modern research, using viruses taken from the bodies of frozen victims, has concluded that the cause of death in these victims was through a "cytokine storm" (over-reaction of the body's immune system). The strong immune reactions of young adults ravaged the body, whereas the weaker immune systems of the elderly, children and immune-compromised resulted in fewer deaths among those groups.

In 1918, there were no vaccines – just palliative care. On the other hand, history reveals that *homeopathic treatment for influenza was very successful*. In fact, homeopathic physicians had much less patient mortality than their allopathic counterparts. For example, one group of 26,795 cases of influenza treated by homeopathic physicians showed a mortality rate of just 1.05%, while that of the average conventional institution was about 30%. Another collection of 6,602 cases treated homeopathically had only 55 deaths showing a mortality rate of .8%.

The same homeopathic remedies still exist!

Medical reports state that homeopathy was 98% successful in treating the 1918 epidemic. Gelsenium and Bryonia were the two most common homeopathic remedies used. Dr. Roberts, a physician on a troop ship during WWI, treated 81 cases of flu on the crossing to Europe. He reported, "All recovered and were landed. Every man received homeopathic treatment."

Warning:

Any treatment recommendations for viruses that produce a "cytokine storm" (overactive immune response) should be approached with caution! This topic will be addressed further in Chapter 8: Chronic infections and "cytokine storms".

Will you survive a pandemic?

The current scare is the Ebola virus. It is rapidly mutating with over 400 strains known at this time. That number may continue to get larger. So the ability of the virus to evolve is faster than the vaccine industry can produce a vaccine based on what is circulating in the wild. You need to think beyond vaccines.

The reason why public health officials are worried about Ebola and similar viruses is the fear that there will be a recurrence of the flu pandemic of 1918 that killed millions of people. It was this same fear that prompted them to release the swine flu/H1N1 vaccine in 2009. That novel flu vaccine was not properly tested for safety or efficacy and contained dangerous preservatives such as mercury in amounts exceeding the Environmental Protection Agency (EPA) recommended safe levels.

It is ironic that the EPA warns us not to eat fish containing high levels of mercury because it can cause neurological problems, but the CDC recommends the seasonal and H1N1 influenza vaccines that often contain mercury. I will not be surprised if the CDC recommends an Ebola vaccine in the near future. That vaccine will also be poorly tested, ineffective and possibly have serious side effects.

Thankfully, a growing body of scientific literature is demonstrating the beneficial effects of nutrition, herbs, vitamins, minerals and homeopathy in the treatment and prevention of viral illnesses. This, along with good common sense, is my reason for writing this book.

So, why do some people survive pandemics and others do not? Dr. Brantly, the American physician who was given an experimental drug when he contracted Ebola, credits his survival to God rather than the drug. In fact, that drug has so far produced a 40% fatality rate in those it was administered to. Would you take a drug that had a 40% fatality rate? This is a drug that is not based on evidence that it even works!

Dr. Brantly not only credits his faith in God but most likely he had a healthy immune system working for him as well. We are born with a blueprint for survival, so it is up to you to give your body the support that it needs to survive.

Somehow, your ancestors survived pandemics, disease, starvation, etc. How? Their immune system kept them alive. You inherited that same immune system! The difference between you and your ancestors is that before World War I, all the food produced in the world was **ORGANIC.** Chemicals had not been created to produce pesticides. Today, we are living in an immune-suppressive environment. You are being poisoned by pesticides, herbicides, GMOs, etc.

And let's not forget about the vaccines. They contain many toxic substances. The 2014 flu vaccine, for example, includes aluminum salts, sugar, gelatin, egg protein, formaldehyde, neomycin and some have mercury. The fine print on the flu vaccine states that it has not been determined if the vaccine even works! What if something goes wrong and a patient has side effects? The vaccine manufacturer cannot be prosecuted! Whoa. Do you want to be a guinea pig?

There are safer options available by supporting your immune system and eliminating immune-suppressive chemicals in your food, water, environment, etc. as much as possible.

Start by having a plan.

The world is closely following what is happening in West Africa. Why are the people there more vulnerable? Poverty, lack of medical infrastructure, unstable governments, fluid borders, lack of rapid testing for infection, outbreaks in crowded cities, displaced refugees looking for food due to inability to harvest, etc.

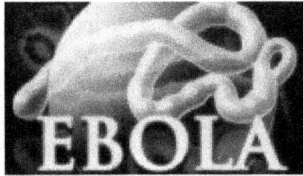

There are many factors that are complicating its containment. With the added benefit of international travel, the genie may get out of the bottle. Although some virologists think it is highly unlikely Ebola could mutate to become airborne, it is not out of the question according to Micheal Osterholm, the director of the Center for Infectious Disease Research. If it does become airborne, even the infrastructure in first world countries could be overwhelmed.

Currently, there are only four hospitals in the US that are prepared for Ebola: St. Patrick Hospital in Minnesota, University of Nebraska Medical Center in Nebraska, National Institute of Health (NIH) in Maryland and Emory University Hospital in Georgia. The total beds for these four hospitals is 11! The bottom line is that health care workers at the inadequately trained hospitals are potentially at risk.

Why is the current epidemic so deadly? Modern research indicates that the Ebola virus creates a deranged, overactive immune response termed "cytokine storm".

This is the same mechanism, coupled with a collapse of adaptive immunity that makes Ebola so deadly. Modern epidemiological research also postulates a past history of tuberculosis or co-infection combined with the particular 1918 influenza strain to greatly increase mortality.

Why is this an important factor in Ebola?

Tuberculosis is endemic to West Africa making it a risk factor. The immune system's inflammatory response is designed to help fight and clear infection, remove by-products, and repair damaged tissue and organ systems. Mostly a protective process, sometimes the failure to return the target tissue to homeostasis can result in destruction.

It is obvious that some people who contract Ebola have an appropriate and balanced immune response that enables them to clear the virus from their system and then mount an appropriate antibody response. Others, tragically, go down the path of "cytokine storm" and die. What's the difference?

Every person's immune system is uniquely shaped by their nutritional status, co-infections (e.g. malaria, tuberculosis), genetic inheritance, gut environment and individual history of previous infections. Other underlying factors include: mode of transmission, age, sex, and immune status. Of course, there is much we do not know yet.

While there is no known effective treatment for Ebola specifically, I think that is because so little attention has been paid to solving this riddle using an integrative approach. No research is currently being done regarding the significance of nutrition, botanicals and homeopathy to target the Ebola virus even though the so-called vaccines are currently not available.

Any treatment of Ebola, beyond supportive measures is an educated guess based on treatment strategies for similar diseases that provoke a cytokine storm such as avian flu, sepsis, certain bacterial infections, ARDS, etc. Strategies in these cases include manipulation of inflammatory cytokines, stimulation of the cholinergic anti-inflammatory pathway, inhibition of COX2 and PGE2, inhibition of Platelet Activating Factor, chemokine manipulation and promoting immune resolution following infection.

There are natural remedies available
to suppress the cytokine storm!

A frequent question asked of me is, "Why do some get the Ebola virus and others do not?" A recent study showed that close to 20% of villagers living in forested areas of Gabon, West Africa had both humoral (adaptive) and cellular (innate) immunity to Ebola making them Ebola-resistant. Another study found that certain people had a genetic mutation that was associated with greater mortality of the virus. On a positive note, research has confirmed that healthy living can effect change in gene expression, essentially reversing the mutation!

In summary, I have seen many viral scares come and go over the years. Usually, they don't live up to the hype and headlines, but you never know what can happen. What I know for sure, however, when it's time for the annual cold and flu season you would be wise to focus on building up your resistance to viruses in general. Ebola or no Ebola, those cold and flu bugs, new ones and old ones, will almost definitely be around and you will likely be exposed.

Chapter 5: Supporting the immune system

People want answers from questions such as: "How can I support my immune system to avoid and/or help my body overcome winter illnesses?"

Some prefer to support their immune system by increasing specific immune-boosting foods alone. Others use supplements, herbs and homeopathic remedies alone. Who is right? Obviously, neither option is right for every individual.

Diet is always the first line of defense for optimal health. Diet is very important because our bodies are chemical factories that make everything they need to remain healthy or to restore health. As fuel, fresh organic food provides the beneficial macronutrients proteins, fats and carbohydrates as well as micronutrients such as vitamins, minerals and fiber. *Food can function as medicine* and minimize the need for supplementation in a healthy individual. I recommend plenty of fresh, in-season produce, especially fruits and vegetables that have high antioxidant and fiber counts. Great examples include *avocado, berries, kale and broccoli.*

Besides a healthy diet, consistent exercise and mindful supplementation, there is a bounty of other lifestyle changes that can benefit immunity that include the following:

- **Maintain good hygiene.** Wash your hands often and keep them away from the face.
- **Don't smoke.** It's a strain on the immune system and the body as a whole.
- **Sleep 7-8 hours per night** to allow the body to repair itself efficiently.
- **Chew your food well** to aid digestion.
- **Drink adequate water** during the day.
- **Lose weight, if needed.** Excess weight can impair the immune response.
- **Herbs and supplements** (discussed later) can improve the immune response. For example, zinc is very important in cases of *chronic* infection/inflammation that depletes zinc stores in the body.
- **Add exercise** to release tension, especially if you have a high-stress job. It works to calm the nervous system by increasing endorphins and neurotransmitters. This in turn, helps the body achieve balance and optimal function, including the immune response.

Exercise can also strengthen the heart which improves circulation, sending more antibodies and white blood cells throughout the body. Thus, the immune system can detect and capture harmful bacteria and viruses more easily.

The rise in body temperature from exercise may also be effective in preventing bacterial growth. In addition, many people report improved bowel function with exercise, which helps to rid the body of toxins.

But *exercise can be a "double-edged sword."* Excessive or vigorous exercise can actually suppress immunity by producing *excess cortisol*. This can make the individual vulnerable to getting sick up to one week after exercise.

Exercise in moderation!

Although the flu and cold season can present us with many challenges, it is not healthy to be afraid. **Fear can also exhaust the immune system**. Instead, I encourage you to focus on gaining the tools you need to succeed in your current environment.

Warning:

The recommendations in this book are not a complete list and some deserving foods, therapies, supplements, herbs and homeopathic remedies may have been overlooked.

In regards to the recommendations for "cytokine storm" and Ebola in this book, I want to emphasize that this is uncharted territory. None of the suggestions listed were studied in human populations with Ebola or highly virulent influenza strains. It is strictly a review of possible therapeutics that *may* inhibit a "cytokine storm" or down-regulate an out of control immune response.

Chapter 6: Disease PREVENTION strategies

Every year from fall to winter, I get many requests for the best natural remedies to prevent cold and flu.

This season, as always, I am recommending the old, traditional remedy - **chicken soup**.

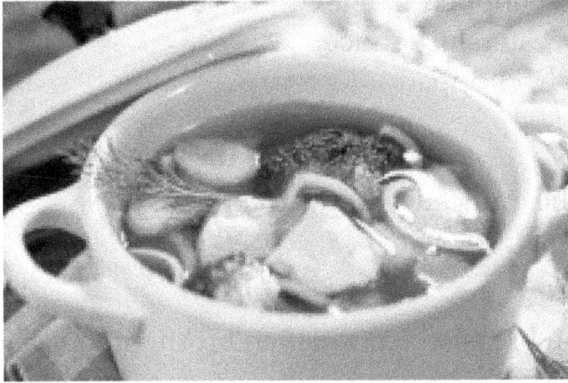

To prevent illness, especially viruses, I absolutely recommend eating good old chicken soup throughout the flu and cold season, particularly if you are exposed to someone who is ill. The recipe on the next page is one of my favorite chicken soup recipes. This "souped-up" chicken soup is loaded with vegetables and spices to support your immune system as well as help thin and expel excess mucus.

Chicken Vegetable Soup

2-3 organic chicken breasts (for extra nutrition, keep bone in)
6 cups low-sodium chicken broth or water
¾ cup short-grain brown rice
1 medium onion, chopped
2 celery stalks, chopped
4 medium carrots, sliced
½ tsp. dried or 1 tsp. fresh thyme
½ tsp. dried or 1 tsp. fresh basil
½ tsp. turmeric
¼ - 1 tsp. cayenne pepper
6 Tbsp. fresh chopped parsley
1 Tbsp. Worcestershire sauce
1 cup broccoli, chopped
1 Tbsp. olive oil
2 tsp. honey
3 cloves garlic, minced
Salt and pepper, to taste

Place chicken breasts, rice, chicken broth, onion, celery, carrots, thyme, basil, turmeric, cayenne pepper, parsley and Worcestershire sauce in a large pot. Bring to a boil and then simmer for 40 minutes longer. Remove chicken, debone and chop into bite-size pieces. Add chopped chicken back into the pot along with broccoli, olive oil, honey, garlic, salt and pepper and simmer for another 30-40 minutes. Serve hot and enjoy! Serves 6.

Mucus – both a blessing and a curse for your lungs.

The lungs produce mucus as a protective agent to trap bacteria, antigens, dust, and other irritants from entering the respiratory passages during breathing. In this way, mucus is a blessing. Unfortunately, one of the symptoms of many common illnesses such as colds, flu, asthma, allergies and chronic bronchitis is the *over-production* of mucus.

Don't ignore the over-production of mucus. The excess eventually gets into the lungs where it can build up and lead to bronchospasms – the constriction of muscles in the walls of the airways.

Coughing is the body's way to rid itself of excess mucus.

But this effort can be challenging when the mucus becomes thick and sticky, leading to breathing difficulties and sleepless nights.

Chicken Soup to the rescue!

More than 30 years ago, Irwin Ziment, M.D., a retired pulmonologist and professor of medicine at UCLA, discovered that ancient healers used natural substances such as *garlic, hot peppers and chicken soup* to address the problem of excess mucus. In fact, he routinely prescribed chicken soup with garlic and hot peppers as a complement to modern drug treatments.

**Treating the bronchospasms without
treating the mucus is backward.**

As he explains it, "Bronchospasm is always accompanied by mucus, but the mucus is largely ignored by doctors. Only the bronchospasm gets treated." It's actually the mucus that's helping to drive the bronchospasms.

How does chicken soup help?

Chicken soup contains a natural amino acid called cysteine (a form of this amino acid, called N-acetyl-cysteine, is a powerful antioxidant that strengthens immunity).

**Chicken soup has been one of my favorite
natural flu and cold solutions since I was a child.**

But it's not enough to just eat chicken soup - you need to spike it with garlic and hot peppers. Why? Because the garlic and hot peppers add heat and pungency - a knockout punch against mucus.

It may sound tortuous but according to Dr. Ziment, when properly prepared, the soup should **_bring tears to the eyes and cause a runny nose as it loosens the mucus_**. I recommend a more measured approach: start with a mild mixture of garlic and hot peppers and work up to a level that you can handle and that is also effective at clearing your sinuses.

A strong physical reaction to the soup means its working!

A runny nose and watery eyes mean the body has been stimulated to loosen mucus at even the deepest levels, making it is easier to cough out the congestion and feel better. There may be no drug or inhaler that can effectively break up mucus in your lungs more than chicken soup. The drugs that affect mucus, such as atropine, merely dry the mucous membranes. And, as the body starts to require the drugs to keep the mucus levels down, a "rebound effect" occurs. Not only does the mucus return when the drugs wear off, it often returns at levels that are worse than they were before taking the drug.

In our pharmaceutically controlled medical system, I doubt chicken soup will ever get due recognition as a standard treatment for respiratory ailments. However, it certainly should be something that doctors recommend. It's natural, nutritious, safe and effective. It can improve digestion, reduce allergies and repair the mucous lining in the small intestine.

It's no wonder that chicken soup has been such a longstanding traditional remedy.

Another nutritious, healthy soup to try is *Mediterranean Vegetable Soup* (gazpacho) prepared mostly with tomato, pepper and cucumber. This delicious soup provides lots of Vitamin C and decreases inflammatory markers like prostaglandin E2. So eat your vegetables!

Why do some people survive pandemics and others do not?

In Africa, for example, *under-nutrition* and nutrient deficiency coupled with chronic infections (parasites, malaria, etc.) can contribute to an ineffective, abnormal immune response.

In the western world, *over-nutrition* in terms of macronutrients of food (corn syrup, simple carbohydrates, etc.), poor quality fats coupled with lack of exercise and micronutrient deficiencies result in the same outcome - immune dysregulation and gut dysbiosis (parasites, bacteria, yeast, etc.).

Lack of adequate vitamins and minerals, especially protein, zinc, selenium, iron and antioxidant vitamins C, D and E, can lead to significant immune deficiency, infections and inadequate cytokine regulation.

Furthermore, under-nutrition in critical periods of gestation and infancy can impair normal immune development.
If the body does not have the necessary building blocks for sustained health, it will break down and not heal properly, no matter how many surgeries, prescription drugs, painkillers or hormones you take.

You don't necessarily need to buy expensive supplements to get all your vitamins and minerals. There is another way. You just need to put aside the *time* to do it.

Think about it. Wouldn't it be great if we could eat a nutrient and have it go to a specific part of the body that needed it the most? Well there is such intelligence in nutrient-dense foods such as

Bone Broths.

Bone broth (sometimes referred to as bone stock) is used in traditional French, Italian, Chinese, Japanese, African, South American, Middle Eastern and Russian cuisines.

Unfortunately, these homemade broths used to produce nourishing and flavorful soups and sauces have almost disappeared from the American culinary tradition.

As a result of our modern meat processing techniques and our hurry-up, throwaway lifestyles, there has been a decline in the use of meat, chicken and fish stocks. In the past, butchers sold meat on the bone rather than as individual filets; whole chickens rather than boneless breasts and whole fish rather than deboned and canned.

There was a time when our thrifty ancestors made use of every part of the animal by preparing stock, broth or bouillon from the bony parts. In fact, bone broth contains the exact minerals, in the proper proportions, that our teeth and bones are made of – 65% Calcium and phosphorus. By stewing bones for several hours or days, the stock becomes very rich with minerals. The bones become so soft that you can push your thumb nail into them. This tells you that the minerals that were in the bone are now in the bone broth.

Bone broth also contains bone marrow where both red and white blood cells are manufactured. Modern science has also discovered that high concentrations of *stem cells* are found within bone marrow. Stem cells influence genetic material and help our bodies build and repair cells.

Why is this important? Our modern diet is sorely deficient in valuable vitamins and minerals needed to support a healthy immune system.

In addition, many people use antacids and acid-stoppers like Prilosec, Nexium, Tums, etc. that interfere with mineral absorption.

And there's more - stomach acid is your main defense against bacteria, viruses and fungus that may enter the oral route. So when you take antacids or acid-stoppers, you will be more vulnerable to infection via the mucous membranes and the gut. There are many natural solutions for acid reflux and indigestion using herbal teas, enzymes, and changing the diet/lifestyle.

Fish stock, made from the carcasses and heads of fish, is especially rich in minerals, including all-important iodine to nourish the thyroid gland. Ancient texts report that fish stock helped patients feel younger and gave them more energy as well as restored their mental abilities. According to some researchers, at least 40% of Americans suffer from low thyroid function (hypothyroidism) with its accompanying symptoms of fatigue, weight gain, frequent colds and flu, inability to concentrate, depression and a host of more serious complications like heart disease and cancer.

You would do well to include fish broth or any bone broth in the diet as often as possible.

How long can bone stock be stored? Clear stock will keep about five days in the refrigerator, longer if re-boiled, and several months in the freezer. It may be convenient to store the stock in pint-sized or quart-sized containers so that you can have appropriate amounts on hand for sauces and stews. If you have limited space in your freezer, you can reduce the stock by boiling it down for several hours until it becomes very concentrated and syrupy. This reduced, concentrated stock, called demi-glaze, can be stored in small containers and easily thawed. Add water to the thawed demi-glaze to turn it back into stock. Be sure to label the kind of stock/demi-glaze that you are storing because they all look alike when frozen.

Bone broth is an invaluable resource for making Chicken Soup and other hearty soup recipes like Mediterranean Vegetable Soup (gazpacho) and Minestrone Soup (recipe below).

Minestrone

2 quarts beef stock
2 carrots, chopped
1 clove garlic, peeled and mashed
1 cup fresh spinach or chard, chopped
2 cups cooked kidney beans
Sea salt and pepper to taste
1 cup rice pasta, broken in bits
Grated Parmesan cheese to garnish

Bring stock to a boil and skim fat off the top. Add remaining ingredients and simmer about 10 minutes. Enjoy!

Bone-Vegetable Broth

Bones (see bones footnote on page 145), preferably organic, free-range and/or grass-fed animals
7 carrots
1 large onion
1 small bunch celery
¼ cup apple cider vinegar
1/3 bunch parsley
salt and pepper to taste
1 large handful spinach
spices: turmeric, thyme, bay leaf, etc. to taste

Fill a large crock pot or stock pot half-full of bones from chicken, turkey (see poultry footnote on page 145), beef (see beef footnote on page 145) and/or non-oily fish (see fish footnote on page 145) bones. If using beef bones, roast beforehand for 25-30 minutes at 375 degrees F and then use them to make a stock. Finely chop vegetables and add to the pot. Cover with cold, filtered or distilled water (distilled water helps to leach the minerals into the broth) (see water footnote on page 145). Liquid should come no higher than within one inch of the rim of the pot to allow for expansion during cooking. Add vinegar to help draw out the nutrients from the bones.

Bring to a boil on high heat and skim off the scum and impurities as they rise to the top. Add spices (tie together if fresh). Reduce heat, cover and barely simmer for at least 4-24 hours or as long as 72 hours for beef broth. The more it cooks, the more minerals will be leached from the bones and vegetables. Skim off the froth as it arises. Add water as it evaporates.

Remove carcasses with tongs or a slotted spoon and strain the liquid into storage containers for storage. Chill well in the refrigerator and remove any congealed fat before transferring to the freezer for long-term storage.

Include the following disease prevention foods:

High quality fats, especially EPA and DHA from cold-water fish such as salmon, flax and products from grass-fed animals that can reduce inflammation. Research reveals that meat and dairy products from grass-fed animals can produce 300-500% more of the anti-inflammatory Conjugated Linoleic Acid (CLA) than those of cattle fed the usual diet of 50% hay and silage and 50% grain. Eggs from CLA-rich, cage-free chickens are also beneficial.

Here's a fact that will surprise many people: research also shows that in order to ward off illness, **50% of the diet should be high quality fats**! Are you worried that eating fat will make you gain weight? Well, if you get half your calories from fat, 30% from protein and 20% from high-quality carbohydrates like vegetables, tubers and berries, you are essentially eating a Paleo diet. Many people find the Paleo diet to be very satisfying and they actually LOSE weight while eating it because the high fat content helps them eat less overall (fats evoke satiety and raise leptin levels). There is an abundance of information about the Paleo diet online and in books.

The remainder of your calories would come from the following:

- Proteins: lean meats, kefir, yogurt, beans, etc.
- Vegetables: dark leafy greens, broccoli, cauliflower, Brussels sprouts, cabbage (any vegetable except corn)
- Tubers: sweet potatoes, carrots, celery, turnips, beets, rutabaga, potatoes, etc.
- Fruit (limit 1-2 per day): berries, apples, etc. (any fruit except oranges)
- Whole grains (gluten and corn-free) such as quinoa, millet, oats, rice, buckwheat

Keep in mind that calorie needs will be different for a 110 pound sedentary female than for an active 250 pound construction worker or a 150 pound nursing mother. Do the math for yourself. There are free calculators online or apps for your smart phone that are able to track your calories and nutrient ratios.

What does a high fat diet look like?

A fat gram is equal to 9 calories per gram, so for a male needing 1800 calories per day, 900 calories should come from fat spread over the day. You could achieve that by eating the following functional foods made up of mono, poly and saturated fats:

½ medium avocado

1 wild Alaskan salmon burger

¼ cup walnut halves

1 Tbsp. chia seeds

5 ounces turkey breast with skin

1 Tbsp. flax oil added to fruit smoothie

1 Tbsp. olive oil in salad dressing

2 hardboiled eggs (with yolks)

1 ounce of 70% dark chocolate

Eat an Anti-Bug diet that includes the following:

Get adequate protein. One in four bites should be good protein sources such as chicken, eggs, fish, beef, quinoa, nuts, seeds, sprouts, etc.

Avoid excess dairy products that can cause mucus buildup.

Eat plenty of vegetables, good fats and garlic to benefit your immune system.

Avoid sugar, processed and junk food. Sugar inhibits phagocytosis, a process in which viruses and bacteria are destroyed by white blood cells. As an example, when you drink a can of soda that contains approximately 9 teaspoons of sugar, the immune system is suppressed by 30% for 3 hours.

Minimize, if not eliminate alcohol and caffeine consumption – they can deprive the body of protective nutrients and can suppress white blood cell activity.

Eat chicken soup frequently, particularly if you come down with signs of a cold or flu.

As I stated previously, chicken soup is a great immune booster; even more so when reinforced with ample garlic, a natural antibiotic and antiviral remedy that has been used worldwide for centuries.

Seaweed is a source of more than 50 minerals. In fact, it has a higher concentration of magnesium, iron, iodine, and sodium than any other kind of food. Seaweed can be added to soups to give extra flavor. Wakami, nori, and kombu are a few seaweeds you might want to give a try.

Blood sugar regulation for a healthy immune response

There is an epidemic of insulin resistance and diabetes in the U.S. due to *over-nutrition*. Normalizing body weight, especially reducing abdominal fat, is an important part of maintaining a healthy immune response since the *major source of inflammatory cytokines is fat* in the body.

Excessive fat mass is associated with over-expression of inflammatory markers. A person who is overweight AND diabetic has chronic inflammation, excessive cytokines and poor immune response to infection.

Studies have shown that obese persons have a greater risk of death from infection with pandemic H1N1 influenza A virus. Diet can go a long way to normalizing blood sugar via a reduction in the amount of simple carbohydrates that most Americans eat.

Get Moving!

Don't just exercise for an hour at the gym 3 times a week. Move all day long. Download a timer for your computer desktop and set it to ring every 20 minutes so you can get up and stretch/walk for a minute.

Lose weight.

Even losing 3-5% of your total body weight can have a huge impact on your blood chemistry.

Optimize gut flora.

Most chronic disease originates in your digestive system. One of the most beneficial steps you can take to improve your health is to maintain a healthy gut. Intestinal bacteria (flora) contains tens of trillions of microorganisms that have a direct impact on health.

For example, it helps the body to digest certain foods that the stomach and small intestine have not been able to digest and it plays an important role in the immune system, performing a barrier effect. Gut flora can be optimized with fermented foods like yogurt, kefir, tempeh, natto, miso, sauerkraut and pickles. Or, you can simply take a probiotic supplement, especially after antibiotic use.

Eat your broccoli!

Researchers at the Linus Pauling Institute at Oregon State University have discovered that the "sulforaphane" compound in broccoli and other cruciferous vegetables such as like Brussels sprouts, cabbage and cauliflower is so good for you that it provides immune modulating effects to prevent cancer - it increases the white blood cell count via increased bone marrow activity. This in turn results in increased levels of infection-fighting antibodies and lower inflammatory markers.

Spice up your immune system.

Don't forget about the preventive ability of spices in your kitchen pharmacy!

- **Rosemary and Basil** have antiviral, anti-bacterial, anti-inflammatory and anti-tumor properties. These spices also enhance digestive function.

- **Curcumin**, the active part of the popular Indian spice Turmeric, has anti-inflammatory and antioxidant properties in many diseases. In a study, researchers injected mice with curcumin 5 days before inoculation with a virus and daily afterwards. The results revealed that curcumin helped to mount an initial inflammatory immune response to the virus and also helped to down-regulate the response at the appropriate time to prevent a cytokine storm. Unfortunately, humans do not have the five-day advance knowledge of exposure to a virus so they can start taking curcumin. Thus, it would be a good idea to add this cooking spice to your food as much as possible (or take a curcumin supplement) during the flu and cold season, especially since it has a long, safe history of daily use for various problems such as arthritis, asthma, diabetes, etc.

- **Ginger** can be used as a spice, a tea or a supplement. It has anti-inflammatory and antioxidant abilities. In fact, simple ginger extract proved as effective as a conventional drug for suppressing inflammation in ulcerative colitis.

- **Parsley** is a cleanser for the glands, liver and gallbladder. It contains lots of vitamins A and C, antioxidants, selenium for use as a natural disease barrier, silicon for tissue repair and zinc. Parsley is also a natural antihistamine!
- **Thyme** can be used as a bronchial dilator to rid phlegm and congestion from the lungs.
- **Sage** is a natural antibiotic, aids in digestion and relieves gas.
- **Garlic** has had a long history of use as a natural antibiotic, antiviral and antioxidant for thousands of years. It can be eaten whole, in food or as an oil.

Include the following lifestyle factors for disease prevention:

- **Manage Stress**. It is our choice how we respond to stress. If prayer and meditation is not your thing, then many creative hobbies can help manage stress. Even observing clouds outside your window can change your mindset.

  For example, knitting, woodworking, quilting, etc. can also evoke the relaxation response to lower heart rate, blood pressure and boost mood. Connection with nature in some way is preferable to being a "couch potato".

So, turn off your TV or computer and get outside every day without sunscreen for at least 15 minutes to get your dose of Vitamin D.

We all have stress in our lives. We just need to find ways to defuse it. If everyday stress becomes chronic, the stress hormone cortisol is over-produced, resulting in the failure to appropriately regulate inflammatory responses in the body. Emotional conflicts such as worry, anxiety, anger, depression, etc. can effectively drain the immune system and leave you more vulnerable to infection.

- **<u>Adequate rest</u>**. Your immune system operates on cycles of rest and activity. Too much activity and not enough rest is a ticket for trouble along with weakened resistance. Many studies show that not enough sleep suppresses the immune system and undermines your ability to fend off infections.

- **<u>Wash your hands</u>**! Good sanitary habits are important. Pathogens are everywhere and hand washing is an important way to prevent getting sick and spreading germs.

I suggest spraying Smart Silver (described later in the supplement section) near the nostrils and into the throat to zap micro-organisms present in these common entrances to the body.

- **<u>Water is essential for good health</u>**. Stay hydrated. Your body depends on water for survival. Did you know that water makes up more than half of your body weight? Every cell, tissue and organ in your body needs water to function properly. For example, you need water to maintain body temperature, remove waste and lubricate joints. It is a fact that many people suffer from constipation simply because they are dehydrated.

How much water should you drink each day? There are different recommendations for water intake but most people have been told they should drink 6-8 glasses of water each day. Since everyone is different, my recommendation is to drink 1 quart of water per 50 pounds of body weight up to 3 quarts per day. Of course, more water intake may be required in hot weather, with heavy exercise, pregnancy, nursing mothers or in cases of fever, diarrhea and vomiting.

A good test for adequate hydration is to check your urine.

You are probably well hydrated if it is consistently colorless or light yellow.

- **<u>Get some sunshine</u>** (or supplement with Vitamin D3). Your bare skin has the natural ability to convert sunlight into vitamin D, a critical hormone-like substance that, among many other benefits, exerts a role in maintaining immune system effectiveness and protection against infections like the common cold, flu, and pneumonia. Fall and winter, however, mean less available sunlight, particularly in the northeast.

Researchers studied data from the 1918 Flu pandemic and saw a correlation between deaths from the flu/secondary pneumonia and the time of year. What is interesting about this research is the finding of reduced mortality in the summertime, a time when people had access to more sunlight.

No matter where you live, make an effort to get out in the mid-day sun (10am to 2pm) for 20 minutes or so to stoke your vitamin D supply.

Some people also supplement with 2,000 IU of vitamin D3 per day during the fall and winter seasons for extra insurance (depending on where you live, time spent in the sun, constitution, diet, etc.).

- **<u>Don't fall into the antibiotic trap</u>**. Too many people do. They run to their doctor and ask for an antibiotic at the first sign of a cold or flu. Colds, the flu, most sore throats, and bronchitis are caused by viruses – they invade healthy cells, multiply and spread.

Antibiotics Do Not Fight Viruses.

Worse, they can increase the risk of a resistant infection down the road and set you up for another bout of illness. In addition, antibiotics can deplete the very important "friendly" gut flora (bacteria) that reside in your intestine and form a major element of your immune system.

- **<u>Take a digital holiday.</u>** This means no Smartphone, television, iPod, computer, etc. We live in an electronic era. The average adult currently spends half their day in front of a screen of some sort. This can lead to insomnia, stress, eyestrain, headaches, anxiety, depression and much more.

A digital holiday will free up more time to get some exercise, plan a healthy diet strategy, talk to someone you love in person, write a letter or just do nothing!

In an era of information overload, always being available, social media, and internet addiction, taking a digital holiday may be difficult for some people because being connected around the globe is such a thrilling experience for them. But it can be unhealthy if not kept in balance (addictive). We risk being "connected" to networks and devices rather than to the people immediately around us.

If a digital holiday is not convenient for you, perhaps something as simple as silencing your phone, putting down the iPad or looking away from the computer screen or television when someone is talking to you could serve the same purpose.

We all need to make time for a Digital Holiday.
Disconnect to reconnect,
and remember what it means to simply be human.

- **<u>Reduce inflammation by reducing body fat</u>**. This can be harder said than done for certain people who have "leptin resistance". Researchers discovered the "satiety hormone" called leptin in 1994 - a protein that is made in the fat cells, circulates in the blood and goes to the brain.

It is the way your fat cells tell your brain that you have enough energy stored to function normally. So when you decrease energy intake (less exercise) and/or lose weight (diet/illness), then your brain senses starvation and increases leptin levels so you are hungrier. The problem is that overweight people have plenty of leptin to shut the hunger signal off but their brains aren't getting that signal to stop eating (leptin resistance).

In other words, the brain is starved while the body continues to gain fat. Why is this? Researchers believe that when the leptin levels are low, food is even more rewarding. When the leptin levels are high, the reward system and hunger is extinguished and food doesn't look as enticing.

But in leptin-resistant people, the reward system doesn't cue a person to stop eating when leptin levels rise. They feel hungrier and the reward doesn't get extinguished.

So they eat more and it becomes a vicious cycle - resulting in obesity. Another very important function of leptin is to keep the immune system happy. Inadequate leptin signaling contributes to chronic inflammation and subsequent immune dysfunction. Scientists are also finding an association between leptin and infertility as well as certain cancers.

Leptin in a pill will not help. It's made by fat tissue and as you increase fat, you make more leptin. It makes no sense to give people leptin if they have an impaired response (leptin resistance). No amount of leptin is going to overcome that resistance. Rather than taking supplements that haven't been proven to help, the following options may help to restore leptin balance:

- o **Get adequate sleep.** Leptin is reduced with sleep deprivation. Keep your bedroom cool, dark and free from electronic devices like cell phones, computers, TV's, etc.
- o **Be careful of fad diets** that trigger the adaptive response to starvation and a decrease in leptin.

o **Increase fiber consumption** (vegetables, fruits, legumes, nuts, seeds). Reduce refined, processed, and fast foods that tend to be high- glycemic and inhibit leptin.

Remember this:
Insulin resistance generates leptin resistance.

So get your insulin down and the leptin will follow. The best way to reduce insulin is through diet. We are overdosed on sugar and carbohydrates in this country. I believe that if the diet is improved, insulin resistance could easily be reduced resulting in loss of fat and inflammation.

One of the hallmarks of insulin-resistance is high serum triglyceride levels – fat in the blood. Triglycerides seem to block leptin transport into the brain (brain starvation). The natural way to reduce triglycerides (no pharmaceuticals, please) is to reduce insulin-resistance, carbohydrates, sugar and get some exercise!

In summary, our best defense against preventing disease is a strong immune system and clean internal/external environments. Proper diet and lifestyle is a must! Regularly consume whole, low sugar foods, exercise in moderation, reduce stress and get sufficient rest.

Include the following supplements for disease prevention:

Vitamin D3 is not only antimicrobial but reduces the production of inflammatory cytokines. As a preventive measure, I suggest that people take a Vitamin D3 supplement in the winter months. The supplement you choose should include Vitamin K2, if possible, to help regulate the usage of Vitamin D in your body.

Most people find that 1,000-2,000 IU of Vitamin D3 is sufficient, but depending on your latitude, time spent in the sun, constitution, diet, etc., you may need more or less.

If digestion is poor, I recommend a liposomal Vitamin D3-K2 supplement that uses a carrier protein to bypass the digestive process and escort the Vitamins D3 and K2 directly into the blood.

An excellent product that I often prescribe to patients is *Liposomal D3-K2* from Desbio. NOTE: Taking mega doses of Vitamin D3 can be toxic (50,000 a day for example).

Colostrum was found in research studies to be three times more effective in preventing flu than the vaccine alone!

Colostrum contains secretory IgA (SIgA), the primary immunoglobulin responsible for immune protection in the gut. SIgA is also important for *down-regulation of inflammatory cytokines*, neutralizes viruses and bacteria, activates an underactive immune system to fight disease-causing organisms and suppresses an overactive immune system (i.e. autoimmune conditions and "cytokine storms").

What is colostrum? It is a non-milk substance produced by the mammary glands of all female mammals (including humans) during the later months of pregnancy to protect the newborn against disease.

Colostrum is 50-60% protein, 30-40% of it consisting of five immunoglobulins that are powerful weapons against disease, especially viral and fungal infections.

It is also rich in vitamins and minerals, including Vitamins A, C, D, E, B1, B2, B6, B12 and folic acid along with the minerals iron, magnesium, zinc, copper, selenium and phosphorus. Another impressive fact about colostrum is that over 37 different immune factors are found in it!

The supplement that I recommend to patients is *Bovine Colostrum* from MarcoPharma for various health concerns including a compromised immune system.

Curcumin, from the spice Turmeric, can be included in your diet every day to prevent seasonal illness. Research has repeatedly shown that Curcumin has a wide and powerful inhibiting effect on many types of microbes, including influenza viruses.

As a dietary alternative, many people prefer to take a daily supplement of 250mg. Increase the dose to 1,000mg if you are coming down with a viral infection.

Echinacea is the #1 preventive, immune boosting herb to take during the cold and flu season. It can be taken daily. Echinacea is known to stimulate production of white blood cell "killer" cells and regulate red blood cells. It's a lymph system cleanser, tumor-inhibitor and is anti-allergenic.

Echinacea tea is a standard for infections *at onset* to stimulate immunity and recovery. Viruses (including the cold and flu virus), gland swelling, lymph congestion, boils, abscesses, inflammatory conditions, and immunity that is compromised by prolonged illness, surgery, or rounds of antibiotics tend to respond well to Echinacea.

I recommend the use of teas as much as possible. The warm water of the tea releases the properties best! A tincture with alcohol just doesn't compare. Please note the following standard for taking Echinacea:

ONE MONTH MAXIMUM, ONE MONTH BREAK.

Monthly breaks let your body's own immune responses show their new strength.

One cup of tea per day is a moderate and effective dose, but many herbalists recommend up to 3 cups of tea per day for a more potent remedy.

If you take 3 cups of tea per day, it's best to take a break from Echinacea after one week and if you need to resume for another week, scale down your use to one cup per day. Echinacea cleans the blood, kidneys, lymph system and liver, protects healthy cells against decay and fights invaders including bacteria, viruses, fungus and microbes. It also stimulates the production of T-cells, antibodies and interferon, is anti-allergenic and anti-inflammatory.

Smart Silver is patented and proven in over 180 scientific studies to destroy bacteria, viruses and fungi. As an alternative to antibiotics, it is safe to use, has no side effects and it does not destroy good, "friendly" flora (bacteria) in the gut. It can be used in every orifice of the body and can be taken throughout the cold and flu season for prevention.

The recent increase in infections due to bacterial resistance to antibiotics is becoming alarming. If a colony of bacteria is treated with an antibiotic that kills nearly all the bacteria but fails to kill all the mutants, those surviving bacteria can multiply and pass on their immunity to new colonies of antibiotic-resistant bacteria.

Not so with Smart Silver.

Why is Smart Silver different?

By teaming with doctors, scientists, independent laboratories, major universities and health consortiums throughout the world, Smart Silver was created with an in-depth understanding of bacteria and pathogenic organisms.

It is not colloidal silver. Smart Silver is manufactured in a patented process utilizing 10,000 volts of electricity that energizes the entire water-base. Therefore, it does not deal with infection on merely a chemical level, as do colloidal silvers, but also works on a measurable energetic level. Many independent studies have been successfully performed against the deadliest bacteria on the planet and certify that Smart Silver is completely non-toxic.

In fact, Smart Silver was tested by medical doctors as a humanitarian effort in one of the world's most bacteria-ridden environments – Ghana, West Africa. Its success as an alternative to antibiotics has given new hope for people in this area.

Smart Silver Uses

- Antibiotic
- Antiviral
- Antifungal
- Analgesic (pain)
- Anti-inflammatory

Recommended Dose:

1-2 tsp. liquid daily

It can also be used as a spray mist (put liquid in a small spray bottle) – spray in throat for sore throat, ears for earache, nose for sinuses, etc.

Some people with respiratory issues breathe in the mist hourly when they are in risky public locations such as a hospital, doctor's office, airplane, etc.

AVOID the following foods for disease prevention:

Refined, processed and fast foods that contain artificial colors, dyes, sweeteners, flavors and texturizers can decrease immunity and increase risk for a body's susceptibility to illness. Examples are white bread, instant potatoes, white rice and refined sugars. These are also high glycemic-index foods that tend to cause blood sugar imbalances.

Many people are immunocompromised due to **Food Sensitivities and/or Food Allergies**. An *Anti-Inflammatory Diet* (see page 147) or allergy testing may be helpful in these cases.

Aflatoxins, which come from mold that grows on specific foods such as grains and peanuts, can suppress the function of the spleen, an important organ for immune function.

Corn, especially when improperly dried, is particularly susceptible to aflatoxins. Consider reducing or eliminating corn and corn-derived products (cornmeal, corn chips, corn syrup, corn oil, etc.).

Other foods high in aflatoxins include: dried fruit and tree-nuts (pecans, walnuts, pistachios, etc.). Dairy and eggs can also contain aflatoxins due to animals that eat contaminated feed. By avoiding corn, one also eliminates GMO corn consumption which has been shown to harm the gut environment. Most vegetable oils, including Canola, soybean and cottonseed oils are GMO as well. This raises a concern because nuts and seeds are part of a healthy diet. In a perfect world, this would not be an issue. I think the risk benefit ratio is on the side of eating high quality nuts *in moderation.*

Another thing to keep in mind about aflatoxins is that research at Lawrence Livermore Labs showed the chlorophyll in leafy greens like kale, spinach, broccoli, bok choy and chard can neutralize aflatoxins. Use of curcumin from the spice Turmeric can also help protect the liver from aflatoxin damage. So enjoy your nuts with a big green salad and a touch of Turmeric!

AVOID the following lifestyle factors for disease prevention:

Excessive exercise (several hours a day) tends to *increase* cytokines, stress hormones and cortisol resulting in immune depression for 24-48 hours post activity. It is possible that during the time of immune depression, microorganisms, especially viruses, have an increased opportunity to invade the host. For those individuals who perform regular, moderate exercise (one hour per day), the immune system will be temporarily *enhanced* which will protect them from infections.

Poor dental hygiene. It is important to brush and floss your teeth daily. The mucous membranes are the primary route of transmission for most respiratory and sexually transmitted diseases. It has been long known by dentists and cardiologists that poor dental health (i.e. gingivitis and periodontitis) can increase inflammatory cytokines. This can then contribute to chronic low-grade, systemic inflammation and atherosclerosis.

Chapter 7: Acute infection plan

At the first signs of infection (fever, aching, sore throat, etc.), *immediately begin nutritional strategies as outlined in the Disease Prevention Strategies* discussed in Chapter 6, especially chicken soup. If you don't feel well, slow down and REST.

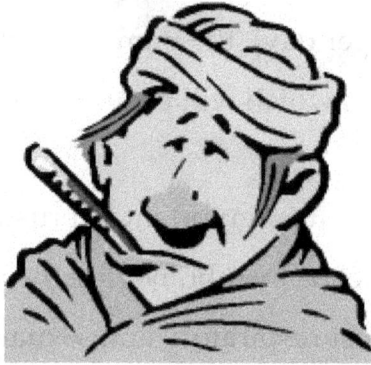

Most people in the U.S. do not have a good diet, which can put their immune system at risk.

Yes, it will cost money to *prepare and prevent*. Everyone has a choice about their priorities.

In this section, I will give recommendations on how to prepare for acute infections *before* and *as* they happen. Modern medicine offers vaccines and antibiotics but in reality, most people around the world still use herbal and homeopathic remedies. Start by expanding your pallet for spices and herbs. Eat basil pesto, turmeric, cumin, garlic, etc. Change what you drink – no sodas, for example! Create a taste for medicinal teas *before* you get ill.

What about fevers?

Naturopathic doctors such as myself, believe that when a fever develops in response to an infection, feeding should be minimal. Chicken soup may be the only thing that can be tolerated because digestion slows down dramatically during a fever. Instead, include water, teas and bone broth as much as possible to avoid dehydration from the increased body temperature.

If diarrhea and/or vomiting is an issue, then electrolyte balance and hydration becomes critical and requires appropriate attention from a medical professional. Supplements should be continued and teas, and/or popsicles/ice chips made from teas are fine.

Most, but not all people can safely fast for 2-3 days when they are ill - discuss this with your health care provider.

Do not suppress a fever with Tylenol or aspirin the first few days.

Aspirin and NSAIDS alone at the initial onset of symptoms was shown in studies to increase mortality by blunting the initial innate response to infection and down-regulating the healthy fatty acids (Omega-3 and Omega-6) that act as messengers for the central nervous system to control the inflammatory pathways.

In the first few days of infection, you want to *enhance* the fatty acid reaction rather than suppress it. Therefore, aspirin and NSAIDS such as Ibuprofen are not recommended in the initial days of infection. In place of aspirin and NSAIDS, begin supplements as outlined in this chapter (if you are comfortable with this approach). Choose only two or three herbs from the botanical list. First, it can be unnecessarily expensive if you take more than 2 or 3 herbs at a time and it may result in overstimulation of the regulatory mechanisms of the immune system.

What if the fever does not go down in a few days?

Fever is a sign that your immune system is responding to an infection. Initially, it is a helpful response that triggers increased production and activation of white blood cells and supports infection fighting immunoglobulins. After a few days, the fever should subside and the resolution phase ramp up.

But in some viral infections, chaotic behavior of the immune system ensues - the fever continues or goes higher, more inflammatory cytokines are made and organ and vascular damage begins.

It is this stage when aspirin, NSAIDS or herbs with the ability to down-regulate the immune system can be helpful.

Bovine Colostrum may be an even better alternative than aspirin,

especially in the elderly population where there is increased risk of side-effects.

Caution should be taken with systemic corticosteroids / Prednisone. Studies have shown an increased death rate from viral infections while taking steroids since this drug depresses the immune response, leaving one vulnerable.

What to do if you START to have symptoms:

Teas, herbs/spices and inhaling essential oil vapors is a good start. For additional safeguards, many people add the following recommendations when they begin to have symptoms of cold or flu:

If you have been taking a Probiotic, Vitamin D3 and Smart Silver as a preventive measure, then DOUBLE the doses.

Otherwise, start taking the following:
- **Probiotic** - 2 times per day
- **Vitamin D3** - 2,000 IU, 2 times per day
- **Smart Silver** - 2 tsp., 2 times per day

Consider adding the supplement **Androgranphis Plus** from Metagenics for additional help to wipe out a virus before it can take hold. Androgranphis Plus is used *short-term* to stop flu, cold, sore throat, and sinusitis symptoms from progressing to a full-blown illness. Many of my patients have used Androgranphis for years to successfully avert illness when started within 72 hours of symptom onset. The recommended adult dose is:

2 tablets every 2 hours for 12 hours, then 3 per day for 5 days.
(half the dose for children under 12 years old)

Androgranphis Plus combines the benefits of the Androgranphis herb with several Vitamin C-rich fruits to promote healthy immune function. Some research indicates that taking Androgranphis Plus in combination with Siberian Ginseng works better than Echinacea or placebo to improve symptoms of the common cold when started within 72 hours of feeling sick. Other research shows that Androgranphis Plus works about as well as Tylenol in reducing fever and the sore throat of tonsillitis.

You might want to have a good supply of Androgranphis Plus on hand before the flu and cold season begins.

Warning:

Andrographis Plus is safe when used for up to one month. Since it increases the immune response, it should not be used with an autoimmune disorder or if the virus has progressed to a "cytokine storm". Similar herbs like Sambucus, Astragalus and Echinacea all enhance immune function by *increasing* inflammatory cytokine production.

In a normal immune response to infection, an increase in cytokines is helpful in fighting infection. Thus, these herbs may be beneficial for healthy people to take at the *onset* of a flu infection only. Astragalus, in particular, may be associated with increased risk of bleeding and blood pressure lowering effects if taken long-term.

In other words, these herbs are very beneficial short-term but it is not wise to include them in certain viral infections such as Ebola with its runaway inflammatory response ("cytokine storm").

What can you do for "full blown" cold/flu symptoms?

In this case, *continue the previous protocol "What to do if you START to have symptoms"* on page 92 except that Smart Silver should be taken as follows:

Swallow 4 ounces of Smart Silver to stimulate the immune system in a one-time dose bolus.

Then, spray Smart Silver in the mouth and nasal passages every half hour or in a nebulizer for 30 minutes a day.

After the one-time dose, take 1 ounce orally 4 times a day until symptoms resolve. When symptoms of the cold/flu are gone, continue the maintenance dose.

Any age group can take Smart Silver – put it on the skin, in the nose, mouth, ears.

Note about Smart Silver:

You may come across a debate about the efficacy of silver products against viruses. The silver product in question is colloidal silver. There is evidence that colloidal silver can help bacterial infections but not viral infections.

Smart Silver is different – it has a magnetic viral DNA disruptor. Keep in mind that viruses consist of a capsid that contains incomplete DNA segments, each containing a slight magnetic charge. Smart Silver is engineered with an opposite charge that attracts the viral DNA and mechanically interferes with the ability of its DNA to replicate.

Healthy DNA does not contain a magnetic charge and remains unaffected by the charge of Smart Silver. So, *Smart Silver only goes after the bad guys and not the healthy, good guys* in your body!

There are published studies that confirm this claim –

Bactericidal Activity of Combinations of Smart Silver with 19 Antibiotics Against Seven Microbial Strains. A. de Souza, D. Mehta, and R. W. Leavitt.

Silver Sol Improves Wound Healing: Case Studies in the Use of Silver Sol in Closing Wounds (including MRSA), Preventing Infection, Inflammation and Activating Stem Cells, G. Pedersen and K. Moelle.

Homeopathic formulas can be very helpful in fighting viruses.

Homeopathy has been used since the late 1700s and is currently practiced throughout the world. It is based on the idea that the body has the ability to heal itself; that "like cures like". In other words, if a substance causes a symptom in a healthy person, giving a sick person a very small amount of the same substance may cure the illness.

Homeopathic medicine views symptoms of illness as normal responses of the body in its attempts to regain health. In theory, a homeopathic dose enhances the body's normal healing and self-regulatory processes.

Historically, people have used homeopathy to maintain health and treat a wide range of illnesses. It has also been used to treat minor injuries, such as cuts and scrapes and muscle strains or sprains. Homeopathic formulas can contain diluted substances such as influenza to fight viruses.

In my practice, I use various homeopathic remedies for viral infections including the following:

Virus Plus from Desbio (1-10 drops under the tongue, 3 times per day) – includes avian flu, Influenza A and B vaccines for the temporary relief of symptoms related to viral infection including fever, fatigue, muscle aches and pains, swollen glands and headache.

Immune Support from Desbio (1-10 drops under the tongue, 3 times per day; in severe cases, take 10 drops under the tongue every 15 minutes; decrease dosage as condition improves.) - This formula includes homeopathic Bryonia, Gelsemium and other ingredients for the relief of symptoms related to cough, fever, muscle pain, irritated throat, swollen glands, bronchial congestion and ear, nose and throat congestion.

Detox III from Desbio (optional) (1-10 drops under the tongue, 3 times per day) - a comprehensive homeopathic formula for use in a weakened immune system, including frequent and recurrent infections, fatigue and swelling.

Note about Homeopathic remedies: Homeopathic remedies should be taken at least 20 minutes away from food.

**In summary, the following is my *First-Line-of-Defense*
recommendations for symptoms of flu or cold:**

1. **<u>Andrographis Plus</u>** - 2 tablets every 2 hours for 12 hours,
    then 3 tablets per day for 5 days.
2. **<u>Smart Silver</u>** - swallow a 4 ounce bolus (one-time dose) to
    stimulate the immune system; then spray it in the mouth
    and nasal passages every half hour (can also be used in a
    nebulizer for 30 minutes a day). After the 4 ounce one-time
    bolus, take 1 ounce orally 4 times a day until symptoms
    resolve. When well, continue the maintenance dose.
3. **<u>Virus Plus</u>** homeopathic - 10 drops 3 times per day under
    the tongue.
4. **<u>Immune Support</u>** homeopathic – 10 drops 3 times per day
    under the tongue.

Most infections resolve with no further intervention than
using the *First-Line-of-Defense* protocol above.

Unfortunately, not everyone has a healthy immune system.
These people may need additional help recovering from flu
and cold symptoms. Furthermore, not everyone is committed
to diet and lifestyle changes to speed up their recovery. As
soon as they feel better, they go back to their old ways and
end up sick again in a few days (relapse).

The following recommendations deal with long-term, *Second-Line-of-Defense* remedies if the First-Line-of-Defense recommendations do not bring about relief of symptoms within five days:

1. <u>**Baicalin**</u> is the herb I use most often for an infection that goes beyond short-term duration. It contains antiviral, antibacterial, antifungal and potent anti-inflammatory properties to inhibit inflammatory cytokines, nitric oxide and prostaglandin E2 in cases of a "runaway immune response."

2. <u>**Zinc**</u> is very important if an infection progresses beyond short-term. Research shows that using zinc gluconate lozenges, for example, seem to help decrease the duration of the common cold and flu, especially when a sore throat and/or diarrhea is present.

3. <u>**Chamomile, Meadowsweet, Ginger and Willow Bark**</u> are specific herbs that inhibit inflammatory cytokines and can be used if the infection is *not* short-lived. In fact, Willow Bark is the raw product which aspirin is derived from.

Remember, none of these herbs should be used in the initial few days of fever.

To suppress the initial inflammatory response could result in the body's inability to clear the viral infection. However, if a cytokine storm develops, these herbs could be good team players.

There are several options for use of the above herbs: supplement form, teas and herbal combinations.

One particular combination that I frequently recommend is **Tricuramin** from Desbio. This comprehensive formula contains White Willow Bark, Curcumin and Boswellia that address the body's inflammatory pathways to relieve pain and the inflammatory response to infection. Consider these three herbs when symptoms of fever, headache and/or sore throat are present – but *only* after the initial few days of fever.

An **Antioxidant Cocktail** can be used throughout duration and recovery to include antioxidants such as a Vitamin E and selenium, resveratrol, NAC/glutathione and quercetin.

Sinusitis Plus, a homeopathic remedy from Desbio, helps to relieve symptoms from sinus infections, whether acute (from a cold or flu virus) or chronic infections related to allergy symptoms. Studies conducted by the Mayo Clinic found that

97% of sinusitis is caused by three to four different fungi. This formula includes these four different fungi.

Another help for nasal congestion is 1-2 ounces of **Smart Silver** added to a netti-pot without the salt.

Essential Oils can be very powerful

Essential oils are concentrated compounds that are found in the seeds, bark, stems, roots, flowers and other parts of a plant. Once extracted, the oils carry the distinctive scent or essence of their plant. Essential oils can be used in the following ways:

- **Diffused in the air (aromatherapy)** – when we inhale essential oils, they go directly to our brain and provide an immediate therapeutic effect. For example, Cinnamon or Eucalyptus essential oil in a diffuser in the bedroom at night can relieve flu symptoms and respiratory distress.
- **Topically**. Never apply an essential oil directly to the skin – they are extremely potent in the undiluted form. Essential oils are easily absorbed by the skin and can be safely applied if you add a carrier oil such as olive oil.

Warning:

Essential oils may not be safe for oral use. Verify that the essential oil is intended for internal use before ingesting it. Furthermore, pregnant women and young children should not use essential oils unless under the guidance of their health care practitioner.

Candibactrin AR from Metagenics is an essential oil supplement that I recommend to patients for immune support associated with intestinal and digestive problems. This amazing formula contains Oil of Oregano, Red Thyme oil, Sage oil and Lemon Balm oil.

A few of my favorite essential oils for immune support are Cinnamon, Oil of Oregano, Tea Tree Oil, and Peppermint. They are easy to grow but keep in mind that as soon as herbs are harvested, they lose potency.

- **Cinnamon** can be used as a spice in the diet or as an essential oil – inhale drops in steam for respiratory problems and to protect against airborne viruses.
- **Tea tree oil** can be put in a cream and placed outside the nose to prevent viral entry to the mucus membranes. It is a powerful antiseptic and antibacterial essential oil.

Many people use it to treat fungal infections such as athlete's foot and nail fungus.

- **Peppermint oil** is a natural antibacterial/anti-viral that can be taken as a tea or mouthwash, inhaled, etc. Anyone can grow peppermint, even in a windowsill.

- **Oil of Oregano** is a must for every medicine cabinet since it is effective against viruses, bacteria and fungus. This wonderful essential oil has been used for centuries for its cleansing and immune-boosting properties. It can be taken after eating a questionable meal to prevent food poisoning and has historically been used for viral pneumonia worldwide (inhale in a steamer).

Some people successfully apply Oil of Oregano topically on spider bites (it denatures protein in venom bites).

Oil of Oregano directions for use:

Diffusion: Use 3-4 drops in a diffuser.

Internal use: Dilute 1 drop in 4 fl. oz. of liquid (if designated for internal use).

Topical: Dilute 1-2 drops with oil, then apply to desired area. Due to its high phenol content, caution should be taken when inhaling or diffusing Oil of Oregano.

Chapter 8: Chronic infections and "Cytokine storms"

Inflammation is the body's first line of defense against infection or injury, responding to challenges by activating *innate* and *adaptive* immunity responses.

Innate immunity is the non-specific, first responder to infection. It is *short-lived* and does not impart lifetime immunity like adaptive immunity does. Made up of specialized subsets of white blood cells, the innate immunity has many functions including recruitment of cells to infection sites via chemical messengers called *cytokines*.

Adaptive (acquired) immunity is composed of specialized white blood cells called T and B lymphocytes which circulate in blood, lymph and tissue looking for foreign microbes. T-cells activate macrophages and Natural Killer (NK) cells to destroy pathogens. B-cells make immunoglobulins that function as antibodies to help neutralize the microbes.

Pathogens are constantly adapting to be one step ahead of the immune system by evading or suppressing certain aspects.

Many pathogens have developed resistance to drugs like antibiotics and antivirals. In these cases, attention has turned to *immunomodulation* as a therapeutic approach.

Unfortunately, this approach can worsen the outcome of certain diseases that produce a "cytokine storm" (a deranged or overactive immune response to inflammation). For these diseases, it has been proposed that ***down-regulating*** inflammatory immune responses may improve outcome to target the pathogen rather than the host response.

It may be that any highly virulent virus will incite a "cytokine storm" (i.e. Ebola virus) regardless of state of health or supplementation taken in advance of infection. But as research points out, keeping levels of inflammatory cytokines as low as possible is a good plan to maximize your odds of a good outcome.

How can you keep inflammatory cytokine levels as low as possible?

Our health is like an island of stability. The island size is determined by our diet, lifestyle, stress management, exercise, avoidance of toxins, etc.

⬇

Disease or dysfunction is a result of factors that cause your island of health to erode
(poor diet, stress, lack of sleep, micronutrient deficiencies, infectious agents, etc.)

⬇

Leading to a greater likelihood that the infection will not get resolved and we get knocked off our stable island.

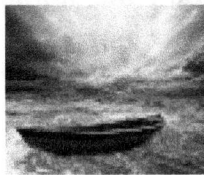

Into the sea of chaos (cytokine storm).

What does a cytokine storm look like?

Generally, a cytokine storm develops 3-6 days after the initial milder onset of symptoms. It includes all the hallmarks of inflammation: redness, swelling, abdominal pain and high fever, along with nausea, vomiting and diarrhea.

Depending on the patient and how the infection has progressed, their temperature may be low. A fast heart rate (greater than 90 beats per minute), breathing rate (greater than 20 breaths per minute) and low blood pressure (systolic less than 90 - that is the first number of the two, e.g. 88 over 60) is also common. To be more precise, laboratory diagnosis via measurements of key cytokines in the bloodstream is required.

A cytokine storm is a medical emergency and necessitates appropriate medical intervention for IV rehydration and supportive care.

What makes a cytokine storm so deadly?

Ebola is an example of a cytokine storm. It can be lethal due to several factors:

1. Damage to liver cells which exacerbates bleeding due to decrease of clotting factors
2. A rapid increase in cytokines and other immune factors that promote inflammation
3. DIC (blood clotting where it should not be)
4. Leaky blood vessels

With a cytokine storm, some components of the immune system have forgotten how to turn off and have gone into over-drive making the adaptive immunity collapse.

A study, the largest of this kind to date, looked at blood from 42 non-survivors and 14 survivors obtained during the five outbreaks of the Zaire strain of Ebola. Death was associated with aberrant innate immune responses (cytokine storm) with hyper-secretion of several inflammatory cytokines and suppression of adaptive immune cytokines produced by T-lymphocytes and CD4/CD8 lymphocytes.

What does this study show us?

Inflammatory markers of a cytokine storm and loss of infection fighting white blood cells (WBCs) were found in those who died. On the other hand, survivors had higher levels of *IFN-alpha,* which is involved in the innate immune response against viral infection. In addition, levels of IL-10 were elevated in non-survivors. This cytokine is a major regulatory messenger for turning off the inflammatory response. At death, significant organ damage had occurred or patients succumbed to effects of dehydration or secondary infection.

As I hope you are beginning to realize,

**Simply boosting your immune system in a
non-specific way could result in more harm than benefit.**

Well-nourished, healthy people with a strong immune system are much less likely to contract the Ebola virus than someone who is exposed to unclean water, food, and parasites. One of the reasons the Ebola virus has spread so rapidly in West Africa is that many people already have a compromised immune system. So the goal should be to raise the bar and get your immune system to a higher level.

Strategies to minimize a "cytokine storm"

As previously stated, with a "cytokine storm", some components of the immune system have forgotten to turn off and have gone into over-drive making the adaptive immunity collapse.

So in theory, it is important to support the liver, assist adaptive immunity (increase immunoglobulin production and activate Natural Killer cells and macrophages) and slow down the innate response of the "cytokine storm" (or at least not stimulate it).

If you can lower the levels of inflammatory cytokines using various strategies like diet and supplements, then you can possibly increase the odds that an infection will have a healthy resolution.

Your best defense against inflammatory cytokines is nutrition and specific herbs.

As in the cases of bird flu, swine flu, SARS, etc., currently there is no specific cure for EBOLA available. Therefore, a strong immune system and clean internal/external environments are the key to prevention of any disease.

Proper nutrition is a must!

Consume whole, low sugar foods, exercise regularly, reduce daily stress and get sufficient rest. I also recommend avoidance of immune system destroyers such as processed, GMO-laden foods.

A wonderful study found that carnosine found in **chicken soup** minimized the action of inflammatory cytokines. It is a fact that the curative power of chicken soup has been scientifically validated for some time now.

Bovine Colostrum is highly recommended for those with a compromised immune system.

Vitamin D3 is not only antimicrobial but reduces the production of inflammatory cytokines.

Dietary intake of copper, zinc, selenium, N-acetylcysteine (NAC), cysteine, methionine, taurine, and Vitamin E have been shown to reduce the inflammatory response. NAC, in particular, significantly decreased the mortality in those with chronic infection.

NAC is a stable form of cysteine that survives stomach acid and is a precursor for glutathione, an important antioxidant that neutralizes toxic free radicals created in the infectious process. Along with vitamin C (discussed later), antioxidants have been observed to be significantly decreased in patients entering into multiple organ failure due to free radical damage to tissues.

Zinc is very important for chronic infections and inflammation that can cause zinc depletion.

Resveratrol, found naturally in the skin of red grapes and red wine, appears to have antiviral, anti-inflammatory and antioxidant qualities. It is known to inhibit respiratory viruses like RSV in children (no vaccine for RSV exists), decrease viral replication of several viruses and down-regulate cytokine production. The suggested dose is 250mg daily with food.

Curcumin helps to disable inflammatory cytokines that can wreak havoc on the immune system. Use as a spice or take 250mg twice a day with food.

Omega-3 Fatty Acids (cold water fish and flax seeds) can help to down-regulate the production of inflammatory cytokines.

Baicalin has a wide spectrum of antiviral activity to regulate innate immunity and down-regulate cytokine production.

Boswellia Serrata/Indian Frankincense exhibits anti-inflammatory properties through the inhibition of various cytokines such as TNF-alpha and COX-2 pathways.

Cat's Claw is a potent inhibitor of TNF-alpha as well as antiviral, antioxidant, anti-inflammatory and immune-regulating activities. In addition, it can decrease intracellular permeability that is common in cytokine storm infections. The antioxidant effect of Cat's Claw helps to neutralize free radicals created in the inflammatory process that otherwise could damage healthy tissue.

Selenium. A deficiency in this antioxidant contributes to a higher incidence of viral mutation and depressed immune competence. Selenium also helps the host to resist oxidative tissue damage caused by viral infection.

Marcozyme tablets from Marcopharma or other proteolytic enzymes work to control inflammation by breaking up inflammatory debris.

Yarrow is an herb that stops bleeding (Ebola can involve internal and external bleeding).

Silymarin, the active constituent of the herb Milk Thistle, has a long history of use for chronic liver diseases. Studies show that Silymarin has an antiviral effect as well as its ability to inhibit inflammatory cytokines. Since the Ebola virus is known to kill liver cells, Silymarin may be beneficial in protecting the liver and fighting the virus. Researchers also discovered that Silymarin inhibits genes involved in the inflammatory response as well as suppresses the production of free radicals.

Garlic is a potent herb that adds a powerful jolt of protection to the immune system, killing yeast, fungi, bacteria, and viruses. Plus, it lowers triglycerides. If you don't like the idea of eating garlic every day, you can take an organic, high allicin, garlic supplement - 1,000 mg a day.

Vitamin C is a major antioxidant. In chronic infections and viruses like Ebola with a cytokine storm, the Vitamin C is removed from the body resulting in the breakdown of organs. The mechanism involved in this is currently unknown.

Scientists are familiar with scurvy that evolves very slowly from the gradual depletion of body stores of Vitamin C. The result is a compromised immune system with series of infections that tend to claim the person's life before the extensive hemorrhage that occurs after all Vitamin C stores have been completely exhausted.

Ebola virus and the other viral hemorrhagic fevers are much more likely to cause hemorrhaging before any other fatal infection has a chance to become established. This is because the virus so rapidly and totally metabolizes and consumes all available Vitamin C in the bodies of the victims so that an advanced stage of scurvy is produced after only a few days of the disease.

Intravenous (IV) Vitamin C is very efficient at entering the bloodstream. Oral Vitamin C is not as effective since interaction with body fluids decreases its bioavailability. *Liposomal Vitamin C* is a possible alternative to intravenous Vitamin C. This form of Vitamin C is encapsulated to protect it through the digestive system resulting in greater amounts of circulating Vitamin C without the diarrhea and upset stomach associated with supplemental Vitamin C.

I encourage you to view the video on YouTube called *"Vitamin C: The Miracle Swine Flu Cure"* produced by 60 minutes. It is a story of a dairy farmer in New Zealand who literally came back from the dead. Doctors were all set to turn off his life support. But his family refused to give up and demanded that the hospital give him IV Vitamin C. It turned into quite a battle between the family and the hospital. Suffice it to say, he is alive today, thanks to his loving family and IV Vitamin C that stopped the cytokine storm that was raging within him. Great story!

Vitamin C is a treatment but not a cure because your immune system actually wipes out the virus; the treatment gives the immune system time to do it. The very first symptoms of Ebola are exactly the same as scurvy, which is caused by inadequate vitamin C. Though scurvy is seldom fatal as a primary condition, it also represents only a *partial* deficiency of vitamin C. The body still has a LOT of vitamin C compared to zero, in the case of a cytokine storm such as Ebola.

Absent ANY vitamin C, blood vessels become very weak and start to lose blood; platelets become ineffective and unable to trigger clots.

So death by Ebola is caused by massive internal bleeding and loss of blood which can potentially be stopped simply by taking enormous doses of vitamin C until the immune system succeeds in killing off the virus.

If the disease seems to be winning, then *even more* vitamin C should be given until symptoms begin to lessen. The oral, liposomal administration should begin simultaneously, but the intravenous route should not be abandoned until the clinical response is complete.

AVOID the following during a chronic infection or "cytokine storm":

- Echinacea angustifolia or purpurea
- Astragulus membraneceous
- Sambucus/Elderberry
- Andrographis/Indian Echinacea
- St. John's wort
- Mushrooms like Maitake, Cordyceps, Reishi and Turkey tail
- Colloidal Silver (Smart Silver is okay)
- Systemic corticosteroids

- Aspirin or NSAIDS like ibuprofen in the initial onset. You do not want to suppress the initial inflammatory response as it would slow down your ability to make antibodies and otherwise fight the infection.

Don't get caught up in fear. It's important to maintain your perspective on the situation.

Chapter 9: Healing with herbal remedies

Hippocrates said, *"Thy food shall be thy medicine."* Herbs, as concentrated foods with vital nutrients, vitamins, and medicinal properties, more than fill the bill. In Hippocrates' time, herbs were the official medicines. Throughout the ages, people in every culture have used herbs for their healing benefits in the same way we use garlic for the vital nutrients that it provides.

Fresh herbs often come with a high price tag at the grocery store. Consider growing your own herbs in a garden or window greenhouse for access to fresh herbs year-round at a significantly lower price.

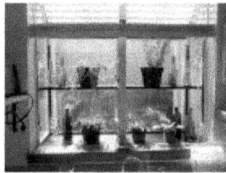

Herbs don't take up a lot of space and easily grow inside or outside with plenty of sunlight. This makes fresh herbs a possibility for anyone, even those without outdoor garden space. It pays off when you can enjoy your own herbs in your favorite foods and teas.

The facts are clear - many bacteria are becoming antibiotic-resistant. Furthermore, antibiotics have no affect against viruses. As you will discover in this chapter, there are many safe herbs that are antiviral, anti-bacterial, antifungal, anti-inflammatory and more.

Guidelines for herbs:

- Herbs should be used as a complement to a healthy diet and lifestyle rather than a substitute.
- Herbs should not be used to replace a doctor's prescription.
- If you are being treated for any illness and are taking prescription medication for that illness, seek your doctor's consent before using herbal remedies.
- Pregnant women, nursing mothers or children should not take herbs without a doctor's consent.
- Do not take a "tonic" herb during a cold or flu.

The healing power of Teas

Teas are an ideal way to get the healing power of herbs into your everyday diet. For example, immunity-building teas can strengthen your own natural defenses or rebuild your strength after antibiotics, illness or surgery. Other teas help with stress and anxiety, tone specific body systems and enhance energy and longevity.

Many herbs have multiple benefits. For example, Chamomile may be taken as a sleep-aid. But it is also beneficial for irritable bowel syndrome, eases indigestion and has antibacterial properties to keep infections away.

Herbal teas are a natural solution for people who want the health benefits of herbs but don't want to take handfuls of herbs as capsules and/or rarely use herbs and spices for cooking.

You can drink herbals teas hot or iced, plain or sweetened. You can prepare them from tea bags or from dried/fresh herbs. Whatever way you prepare the tea, you will be amazed at the potential for drugless healing that is available in herbal teas.

Herbal teas can be used as skin washes or compresses to heal wounds and reduce inflammation since vital nutrients are absorbed through the skin. They can also be used in the bath, inhaled as a steam in a pot of boiling water, etc.

The water used to brew teas make the herbs more effective. Why? Because water, which is essential for the absorption and assimilation of nutrients, diffuses the potency of the herb and delivers its properties in a manner that is harmonious with your natural body processes. Unlike herbal capsules that never touch your taste buds, herbal teas follow the normal digestive process from the mouth throughout the digestive system which is an automatic regulator for substances entering your body.

A standard tea bag contains one teaspoon of a dried herb.

It's a good rule to take teas as needed once or twice a day and use it for one week. After a week, evaluate your progress. If the problem has abated, there's no reason to take the tea every day. Another option is to use the tea intermittently, for a tune-up.

How to use teas:

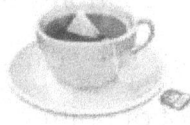

Tea bags are premeasured, quick and easy. Just boil water, pour it over the tea bag and wait 3-5 minutes.

Loose, dried herbs are convenient for herbal combinations. Put a heaping teaspoon in a tea ball or filter and add boiling water; cover the cup and let the herbs steep for 3-5 minutes. Steep the tea a little longer for a richer brew – 10 to 20 minutes.

Fresh herbs from the garden can be frozen or dried for later use. Each herb has specific parts used for their healing properties. Wash the fresh herbs thoroughly before using. Cut the herb into small pieces and *use two tablespoons of fresh herb per cup*. Pour boiled water over the herbs, cover and let stand for 7-20 minutes, then strain.

You can make extra tea and store it in the refrigerator to drink later. It will retain its flavor for up to two days.

Some herbs use the harder parts of a plant such as bark, twigs, seeds and roots which require a longer process. Cut the hard parts into small pieces and place 2 tablespoons of fresh herb per cup into a saucepan with cold water. Bring to a boil, reduce heat and simmer for one hour. Strain and drink. Ginger root is an example of this method.

Examples of herbal blends

The standard dose for a cup of herbal tea is one teaspoon of dried herbs, whether you are using one herb or several herbs. There are many possible combinations. The following are a few of my favorites:

- Rose hips with Echinacea as a cold remedy for its vitamin C and antioxidant power.
- Elderflower, Echinacea, Thyme and Peppermint for flu symptoms – drink it warm if you have chills; drink it cool if you feel feverish.
- Echinacea, Peppermint and Rosemary for bronchitis.
- Echinacea, Elderflower, Ginger or Peppermint and Plantain at onset of colds and congestion.
- Elderflower, Thyme and Peppermint for an antiviral, anti-inflammatory and decongestant.
- Elderflower is ideal for any "itis" condition – sinusitis, colitis, arthritis, etc.

- Dong Quai, Meadowsweet, White willow for inflammation and pain.
- Elderflower, Sage and Thyme for sore throat.
- Cinnamon, Dong Quai, Echinacea and Pau D' Arco for viruses.

Herbal Remedy Descriptions

Baicalin (Scutellaria)

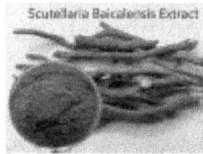

Scutellaria Baicalensis Extract

The process of replication and multiplying of viruses, bacteria and fungi is blocked by the high flavonoids in Baicalin. These flavonoids also *inhibit inflammatory cytokines*.

Some other uses include: cough with thick yellow phlegm, influenza, pneumonia, ear infections, and more. Baicalin is useful in allergies, asthma and sinusitis since it *controls histamine release* upon exposure to allergy triggers. *Skin ailments* such as boils, sores, swelling, eczema and psoriasis also respond well to Bailcalin.

This herb is one of the most respected *nerve tonics for anxiety and stress*. It works by blocking overproduction of stress hormones. Thus, it can be useful during withdrawal from alcohol, nicotine, drugs and tranquilizers.

Baicalin summary of medicinal values: antiviral, antibacterial, antifungal, antihistamine, allergies, skin ailments, anti-inflammatory, nerve tonic for anxiety and stress.

Chamomile

There are many varieties of chamomile but only two are used medicinally – Roman and German chamomiles. A warm tea of chamomile flowers will ease your aches and give you a mellow feeling to lull you to sleep. Chamomile can relieve nausea, stop vomiting, and relieve intestinal spasms, bloating and gas. It has been used through the ages as a bronchial relaxant in cases of asthma, hay fever and sinusitis.

Chamomile summary of medicinal values: anti-spasmodic, digestive aide, anti-inflammatory, sedative, antibacterial, prevents vomiting.

Dong Quai

Dong Quai has a reputation of being "the supreme female tonic" but it is equally valuable for men as well. Another quality that it is known for is to move stagnated body fluids such as blood and redistribute the fluids throughout the body.

Dong Quai contains antiviral, antibacterial and antifungal properties. In fact, a research study showed that it increased survival by 90% when given daily for 5 days at the first sign of infection and continued until resolution. Wow! Dong Quai contains the antioxidants Vitamin E and selenium, which help to build your body's natural barrier to disease. Other minerals include silica for tissue repair, iron for healthy blood, and a wealth of other nutrients to strengthen the immune system.

Dong Quai can stabilize heart irregularities and relax the heart muscle to relieve stress on the heart, probably due to the magnesium, B12 and Vitamin E – resulting in internal tranquility. The zinc and calcium can help to relieve PMS tension and stabilize hormones.

Warning: Dong Quai should be avoided in diabetics.

Dong Quai summary of medicinal values: blood tonic, anti-spasmodic, anti-inflammatory, antiviral, antibacterial, antifungal, digestive tonic, hormone stabilizer; high in vitamins E, A, C and B complex as well as minerals such as iron, calcium, potassium, magnesium, phosphorus, zinc, selenium, and silicon.

Echinacea

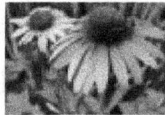

This North American perennial is in many modern herb gardens because of its medicinal value as an immune system beauty. Echinacea is known to stimulate production of white "killer" cells and regulate red blood cells. As a tea, it is a standard at the *onset of infections* to stimulate immunity and recovery of colds, flu, viruses, gland swelling, lymph congestion, inflammatory conditions, and a compromised immunity from prolonged illness, surgery, or rounds of antibiotics.

**The warm water of the tea releases the properties best!
A tincture with alcohol does not compare.**

The standard recommendation for taking Echinacea is:

One month maximum; One month break.

Monthly breaks let your body's own immune responses show their new strength.

One cup of tea per day is a moderate and effective dose.

Many herbalists recommend up to 3 cups of tea per day for a more potent remedy. If you take 3 cups of tea per day, it's best to take a break from Echinacea after *one week*. If you need to resume for another week, reduce to one cup per day.

Echinacea cleans the blood, kidneys, lymph system and liver. It protects healthy cells against decay and fights invaders including bacteria, viruses and fungus by stimulating the production of T-cells, antibodies and interferon. As a bonus, it has health-building vitamins and minerals.

Italian scientists have documented evidence showing that Echinacea protects the skin from oxidative damage from the sun (wrinkles and precancerous growths).

Use the tea as a facial toner and refrigerate the remaining tea for repeated use.

Echinacea summary of medicinal values: immune stimulant, antibacterial, antiviral, antifungal, anti-inflammatory; source of vitamins A, B, C,E and minerals calcium, magnesium, silicon, selenium, potassium and manganese.

Elderflower

Elderflower is known as the "*Chest Remedy*" for upper respiratory conditions such as hay fever, colds, coughs and flu. Taken for a week or two before the pollen count rises can strengthen the respiratory tract and resist allergic reactions. For an extra boost, combine it with the anti-histamine feverfew, which relaxes bronchial muscles to reduce spasms. Elderflower has a long history as a remedy for colds, coughs and flu. Hot tea, in particular, helps to clear the respiratory passages. As a gargle, it can relieve a sore throat and due to its high content of vitamins A and C, can reduce fever and move imbedded phlegm.

Elderflower summary of medicinal values: expectorant, phlegm remedy, fever reducer, diuretic, Vitamins A and C.

Meadowsweet

Meadowsweet is known as the *acid reliever* in cases of acid reflux and digestive distress. It has a soothing mucilage that coats and protects the lining of the digestive tract to restore it over time.

Meadowsweet is also known as *nature's aspirin* due its salicylate content. In the 1890s, Bayer created the synthetic version of salicylates known as aspirin. While aspirin can cause gastric bleeding and gastric distress if it is taken routinely, the natural salicylates in meadowsweet are not known to produce these side effects.

Caution: Avoid meadowsweet if you are sensitive to aspirin or salicylates.

Meadowsweet summary of medicinal values: digestive remedy, fever reducer, anti-inflammatory, diuretic, astringent, anti-rheumatic.

Milk Thistle

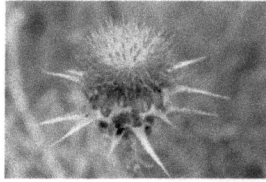

Milk Thistle is a valuable herb to **strengthen your liver**, which can in turn boost your resistance to disease and help you recover from illnesses more quickly.

Your liver plays an important role in immunity. It manufactures chemicals to clean your blood and helps to detoxify your system of harmful chemicals, pollutants, and metabolic wastes. It also secretes bile to stimulate digestive juices so that nutrients from foods can be absorbed.

Many everyday problems are linked to liver deficiency, including recurring headaches, skin problems, depression, poor circulation, chronic fatigue, indigestion, irritability, mood swings, lack of concentration, and diminished resistance to disease.

More advanced liver disorders can result from excessive use of alcohol, drugs, and side effects from medications that cause liver damage.

Milk Thistle is the only known natural compound that protects liver cells and renews liver vitality, even during disease states. If you suffer from depression or recurring headaches due to liver weakness, try Milk Thistle as a routine tea.

This wonderful herb can also be a vital aid in recovery programs such as:

- Withdrawal from alcohol or drugs
- Recovery from the side effects of liver-damaging medications
- Before and after chemotherapy or radiation treatments to insure minimal damage to the liver
- To aid recovery from liver diseases such as hepatitis

Milk Thistle summary of medicinal values: Liver strength, anti-allergenic (decreases histamine), antitoxin, antiaging, antioxidant.

Oatstraw

Oatstraw is a full-body tonic to strengthen your immunity and build your energy. It can help to stabilize thyroid function, regulate blood sugar, reduce cholesterol levels, and bathe the nervous system in nutrients for health and harmony.

It has plenty of antioxidant power, antibiotic properties and it's a natural antidepressant.

Use it as a routine tea to fight exhaustion and fatigue, for recovery from illness, to resist stress, combat anxiety, depression, insomnia and for natural resistance to disease.

Oatstraw summary of medicinal values: antibiotic, antioxidant, antispasmodic, nerve tonic, diuretic, contains vitamins A, D, B1, B2, E and minerals calcium, iron, selenium, silicon, magnesium, manganese, and zinc.

Parsley

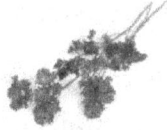

Parsley has been called "The Green Goddess." Grow your own, or buy it fresh. It's a cleanser for the glands, liver and gallbladder, a tonic for the skin, arteries, and capillaries and has mild antibiotic properties to fight infections.

It contains plenty of Vitamins A and C, antioxidants, protein, B-complex, chlorophyll for the cells, selenium for a natural disease barrier, silicon for tissue repair and zinc. *At the first sign of an illness, parsley tea will give you a jump-start to recovery*.

Parsley is also a *natural antihistamine* – great for people with asthma, allergies, hay fever and headaches.

Parsley summary of medicinal values: antibiotic, antihistamine, antioxidant, contains Vitamins A, C, B-complex, along with protein, chlorophyll and minerals selenium, silicon and zinc.

Pau D' Arco

Pau D' Arco is a rain forest herb that has been referred to as a cure-all in Central and South America. It is packed with nutrients including iron, calcium, magnesium, selenium, Vitamins A, C and B complex, manganese, zinc, potassium and sodium. It has antibiotic, antibacterial, antiviral, antimicrobial, antifungal and anti-tumor qualities. The iron in Pau D' Arco helps to build red blood cells and improve hemoglobin production. It's also great for candida control and parasite infections which can compromise immunity.

In the mid-80's, test tube research in Germany showed that Pau D' Arco stimulated macrophages, granulocytes, lymphocytes and T-cells to fortify immunity.

Pau D' Arco tea has successfully been used to fight skin problems such as psoriasis, eczema, ringworm and scabies.

Pau D' Arco summary of medicinal values: antifungal, antiviral, antibacterial, immune stimulant, a source of Vitamins A, C and B complex, minerals iron, calcium, magnesium, selenium, manganese, zinc, potassium and sodium.

Peppermint

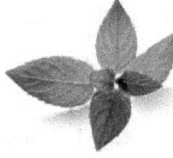

Peppermint is mentioned in the Bible as one of the herbs that was used for paying taxes. In ancient Greece and Rome, it was used to flavor sauces and wines and had a special place in festivals.

The British take their mint seriously and often do what is called "The Peppermint Cure" – drink peppermint water to ward off colds or disease at the onset.

A teabag of peppermint in a pot of boiling water used as an inhalant will ease laryngitis and bronchitis.

Peppermint summary of medicinal values: antispasmodic, immune stimulant, decongestant, tonic, good source of Vitamins A, B-complex, C, and flavonoids.

Plantain

Plantain is one of the finest herbs for general health and **recovery from illness**. It's a decongestant and blood cleaner, it's good for the liver, kidneys and heart and it's the herb to remember when you aren't feeling up to par. It's great for unclogging passageways, particularly lung plugs and liver obstructions (imbedded phlegm). It has been used through the ages for infections in the stomach, digestive tract, bowel, urinary tract and liver.

For fast hemorrhoid relief, take a sitz bath in plantain tea as well as drink the tea. Plantain works as an antidote to venom and poisons, including spider- and snakebites by cleaning toxins from the blood.

Plantain summary of medicinal values: detoxifying, decongestant, expectorant, wound healing, astringent (hemorrhoids), minerals, Vitamins C and K.

Rose Hips

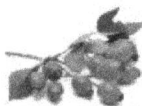

Rose Hips contains many vital nutrients for immunity, longevity and well-being. It's cleansing to the respiratory tract so you can breathe easier; it's a tonic for energy so you tire less easily; it gives disease protection so you aren't as susceptible to colds and viruses.

According to a Christmas legend, the moment the Christ Child was born, every rose in the world bloomed. In ancient Rome, the rose was used as a tribute or blessing. In England, when famine was rampant, rose hips were used for food since it contains various nutrients.

Rose Hips summary of medicinal values: antiviral, antibacterial, antidepressant, blood tonic, antioxidant, kidney tonic, hormone regulator, adrenal support, antispasmodic, anti-inflammatory, digestive aid, phlegm remedy, source of Vitamins A, B complex, C, D, E, K, bioflavonoids, pectin (fiber), and the minerals calcium, iron, zinc, silicon, selenium, magnesium, potassium, manganese, phosphorus and sulfur.

Rosemary

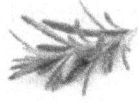

Rosemary has a long history of medicinal use and cooking. It is known to be antiviral, antibacterial and anti-inflammatory to fight infections. It has no side effects and can be consumed regularly.

Rosemary relaxes and tones the nerves, enhances the flow of digestive juices, and improves the body's ability to absorb nutrients. It has been used through the ages to relieve bronchial infections and stimulate blood flow through the heart resulting in improved oxygen to the brain.

Not only is Rosemary a tonic, but it also eases anxiety, depression and tension headaches.

Rosemary summary of medicinal values: antiviral, antibacterial, antioxidant, expectorant, decongestant, circulatory tonic, digestive tonic, antispasmodic, antidepressant, relaxant.

Sage

Sage is called the **longevity herb** because it improves vitality. As an antibiotic, it fights infections and is high in nutrients to tone the body. It is a great stimulant for sluggish livers and associated symptoms such as headaches, fatigue and reduced immunity.

The steam from sage tea water can be inhaled to clean sinus passages. It is also used in respiratory infections such as colds, tonsillitis and bronchitis.

Women often use sage as a reproductive tonic to ease menstrual irregularities and reduce hot flashes in menopause.

CAUTION: Moderate use is best. Avoid sage if you have epilepsy.

Sage summary of medicinal values: antibiotic, antispasmodic, reduces sweating, lowers blood sugar, promote bile flow, sedative; contains Vitamins A, B complex, C, E and minerals calcium, iron, magnesium, manganese, phosphorus, potassium, selenium, sulfur, and zinc, plus flavonoids and estrogenic compounds.

Thyme

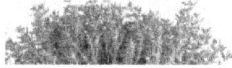

Thyme tea can be a valuable *bronchial dilator to rid phlegm and congestion from the lungs*. Its powerful antiseptic action cleanses the respiratory tract of fungal, bacterial, and viral infections. Begin with a mild tea once a day for a week, then gauge your progress. As you begin to feel less tightness in the chest, you can use the tea less frequently.

A cup of thyme tea can be the tonic you need to make a real breakthrough in colds and flu. It has been effective in urinary tract and kidney infections, even after other methods have failed. Use thyme teas as a gargle for thrush conditions.

One thyme tea bag (or one spoonful of dried herbs) in a pot of boiling water can be used as a steam inhalant for sinusitis due to fungal infestation. You can also use thyme to clean sickroom air by boiling the herb in an uncovered pot on the stove, letting the antiseptic steam purify the air.

Thyme is an antiseptic for all skin infections. Apply the tea topically to increase blood flow to the area and purge infection. Even if the infection is deep-seated, stay with the antiseptic wash until the condition is healed.

It can also be useful as a wash to kill ringworm and thrush in the mouth and throat. Thyme tea has been used to treat fungal infections such as athlete's foot and nail fungus– prepare a tea using 2 tea bags (or 2 teaspoons of dried herbs) and soak feet/nails in the solution until resolved.

Thyme summary of medicinal values: antibacterial, antiviral, antifungal, antispasmodic, bronchodilator, decongestant, antiseptic, expectorant, source of Vitamins C, D, B complex and minerals chromium and manganese.

White Willow

White Willow bark is a **natural anti-inflammatory** herb due to its "salicylic acid" content. It is often found in blends like *Tricuramin* from Desbio for fever, neuralgia, arthritis, rheumatism, bursitis and lumbago. White Willow has also been used as a remedy for chronic diarrhea and dysentery.

White Willow summary of medicinal values: anti-inflammatory, antiseptic, rids worms, source of Vitamins A, B complex, C and minerals calcium, phosphorus, magnesium, manganese, potassium, selenium, sodium, and zinc.

Footnotes

Bones - Ask your local butcher or grocery store for a carcass of chicken or beef bones (many call them "dog bones" or "soup bones"). You can also keep all the bones from the meat you eat during the week in the freezer until you are ready to use them.

Poultry - For chicken, turkey or duck stock, use whole, free-range chicken or 2-3 pounds of bony chicken parts such as necks, backs, breastbones and wings. If you are using a whole chicken, cut off the wings and remove the neck, fat glands and the gizzards from the cavity. Cut the neck, wings and other parts into several pieces. By all means, use chicken feet if you can find them – they are full of gelatin (Jewish folklore considers the addition of chicken feet to be the secret for a successful broth). The skin and smaller bones, which will be very soft, may be given to your dog or cat.

Beef - Good beef stock can be made with several sorts of beef bones. Knuckle bones and feet impart large quantities of gelatin to the broth; marrow bones give flavor and nutrients; meaty rib or neck bones add color and flavor. Lamb and venison can also be used.

Fish - Ideally, fish stock is made from non-oily fish like sole, turbot or rockfish. Oily fish such as salmon can become rancid during the long cooking process. Be sure to use the heads as well as the body – these are especially rich in iodine and fat-soluble vitamins.

Water - Essential to all broths is starting with *cold* water. As the ingredients warm in the water, their fibers open slowly, releasing their juices to add flavor.

Anti-Inflammatory Diet

If you have any type of digestive problem, inflammation, autoimmune condition, pain, etc., the cause may be the foods you are eating.

AVOID the following for 2 weeks:

- <u>Sugar</u> in all forms (this includes honey, maple syrup, molasses, deserts); **stevia is okay**
- <u>Milk</u> (from animals); **yogurt, butter, cheese, and coconut/almond milk in moderation is okay**, *if* tolerated.
- <u>All wheat and gluten foods</u> (wheat, corn, rye, barley, spelt and kamut); **rice, oats, quinoa, millet, buckwheat, amaranth, tapioca is okay**, *if* tolerated.
- <u>Corn</u> in all forms; **all other vegetables are okay**, *if* tolerated.
- <u>Fruits</u> – limit to 1 per day (no oranges)
- <u>Soy and Peanuts</u> in all forms; **other beans, nuts and seeds are okay** in moderation, *if* tolerated.
- <u>White potatoes, tomatoes, peppers, eggplant</u> ("nightshades" can increase inflammation)

- <u>Pork, ham, bacon, shellfish, cold cuts, hot dogs, sausage, canned meats</u>; fish (wild-caught), chicken/turkey/eggs (organic), wild game, lamb/beef (grass-fed) is okay, if tolerated

- <u>Margarine, shortening, hydrogenated/canola oils</u>; olive, coconut, flax, sesame oils are okay, *if* tolerated.

- <u>All sodas, caffeinated teas/coffee, alcohol, all artificial sweeteners</u> (stevia is okay), <u>MSG, processed/fried foods, barbecue sauce, ketchup, chutney, chocolate, mayonnaise</u>; oil and vinegar is okay for salad dressing.

At the end of the two weeks, you may reintroduce **one avoided food every three days**. For example, on day 15 (after 14 days on the Anti-Inflammatory Diet), you might choose to reintroduce milk. Consume 1-2 servings on this day (day 15) only.

If you observe any negative reactions (headache, fatigue, digestive upset, sinus congestion, skin irritation, change in bowel movements, etc.) during the next three days (days 15, 16, 17 in this example), then you must keep this food item out of your diet for at least 3 months and then try again.

NOTE: Some patients with wheat/gluten sensitivity can tolerate sprouted grains.

Breakfast suggestions: eggs and turkey bacon; oatmeal/cream of rice/cream of buckwheat with plain yogurt or kefir and fruit; cottage cheese and fruit; nut butter on rice almond bread; gluten-free burrito with egg, cheese, veggies, salsa (if tolerated); rice protein shake with yogurt and fruit

Lunch/Supper suggestions: large salad with various veggies and acceptable protein above (eggs, meat, fish, poultry, etc.); Baked sweet potato, protein and veggies; gluten-free sandwich with protein and veggies; chicken and/or bean soup and salad; spaghetti sauce (if tomato sauce does not increase inflammation) with meat over spaghetti squash or rice pasta; three-bean salad with grilled salmon and veggies

The 8 Laws of Health

Most people get sick because they violate one or more of the following 8 Laws of Health. There are no shortcuts to optimal health. **You must start with proper diet and lifestyle**.

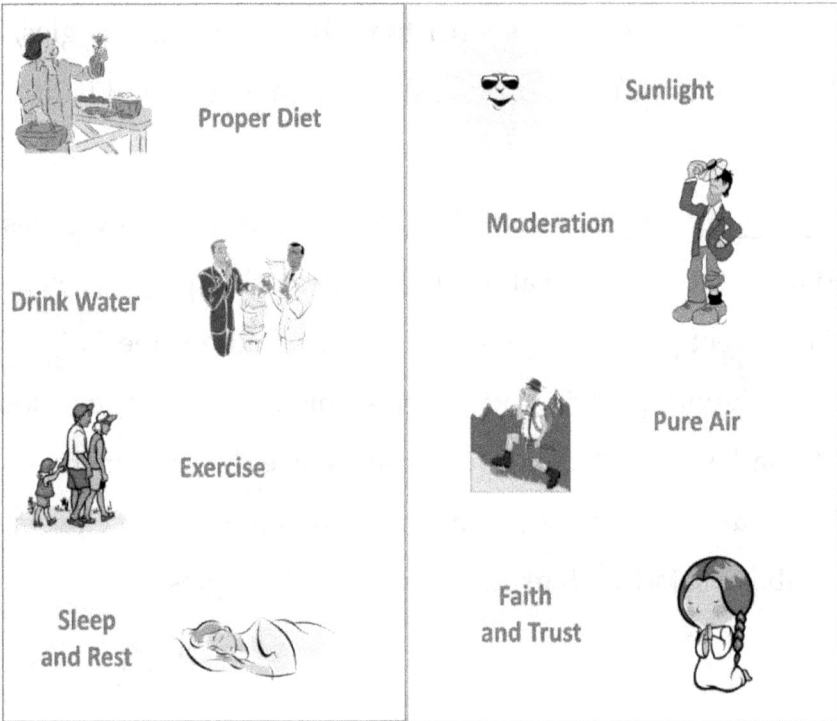

Proper Diet

Sunlight

Moderation

Drink Water

Pure Air

Exercise

Faith and Trust

Sleep and Rest

Unless you have a DIET and LIFESTYLE that supports health, then all the medications, supplements and exercise in the world will not provide what you need to sustain OPTIMAL HEALTH in a simple way.

About the Author

Carol Perkins, N.D., owner of *Natural Choices Clinic* in Lexington, Kentucky, has remained true to the nature of naturopathic medicine, **"Treat the patient, not the disease."**, for 15 years.

Dr. Perkins is a graduate of a four-year accredited naturopathic medical school and a member of the AANP, the national organization for the profession. Her approach to health blends centuries-old, natural, non-toxic therapies with current advances in the study of health and human systems.

Her greatest joy is sharing her knowledge gleaned from research and life experiences as a Naturopathic Doctor (N.D.). People want to know how to stay well in a toxic world. They are searching for answers on the internet, from the media, self-help books, each other and their doctors. But with so much varied information available, who do you trust to give you truth?

Dr. Perkins' intention in her practice and in her books is to inform, educate and inspire people to become active participants in their journey for optimal health and vitality!

She understands that each person' situation is different and a "one-size-fits-all" plan will not work. Nevertheless, she always attempts to direct patients and readers back to simple living using the 8 Laws of Health to keep them on course.

Carol is quite familiar with this simple living concept. She grew up in a very small farming community in northern Ohio. Everyone knew each other and took care of those in need. For their medical needs, they called for "Doc Lewis", the country doctor who concocted his own remedies and made house calls. That was a time when people relied on common sense and wisdom passed down from generation to generation.

Prescription drugs were unheard of back then, vaccinations were minimal, if at all, and gardens and livestock carried them through the years with nutritious, organic food.

Life was indeed simple. The only access her family had to electronics was watching television for one hour on Sunday nights. But it was enough because as a child, it was more important to be playing outdoors and having fun or simply reading a book.

Dr. Perkins believes the simple life is what most people truly desire. The 8 Laws of Health that she often refers to in her books reflect this simple life concept as well as the true path to optimal health!

She has several ideas for future books in the works such as 'How to Stay Young at 100', 'Living the Simple Life,' and '21 Days to a Healthy You.'

Summary of Recommendations

	Prevent infection	Acute Infection	Chronic infection, Cytokine Storm
Optimize diet/lifestyle	√	√	√
Chicken soup	√	√	√
Colostrum	√	√	√
Vitamin D3	√	√	√
Curcumin (Turmeric)	√	√	√
Probiotics	√	√	√
Echinacea	√	√	
Smart Silver	√	√	√
Andrographis Plus		√	
Homeopathic Virus Plus, Immune		√	
Baicalin			√

Thank you for reading my book. I hope it helps you and your family to stay well throughout the year. If you enjoyed this book, please take a moment to leave me a review at your favorite retailer.

Carol Perkins, N.D., Health Coach